ETHICS IN PRACTICE

ETHICS IN PRACTICE

A guide for counsellors

EDITED BY
Kathie Crocket,
Margaret Agee and
Sue Cornforth

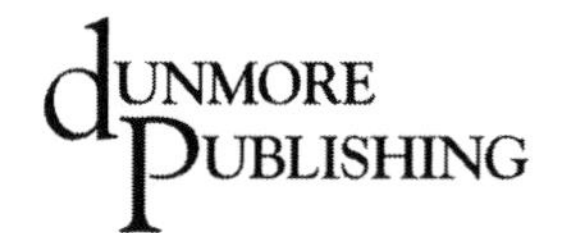

© Kathie Crocket, Margaret Agee and Sue Cornforth

Published in 2011 by
Dunmore Publishing Ltd
P.O. Box 25080, Wellington
books@dunmore.co.nz

National Library of New Zealand Cataloguing-in-Publication Data

Ethics in practice : a guide for counsellors / edited by Kathie
Crocket, Margaret Agee and Sue Cornforth.
Includes bibliographical references and index.
ISBN 978-1-877399-572
1. Professional ethics—New Zealand. 2. Counselling psychology—
New Zealand. 3. Social workers—Professional ethics—New
Zealand. I. Crocket, Kathie. II. Agee, Margaret Nelson.
III. Cornforth, Sue.
174.20993—dc 22

Text: Arno 11.5/13.8
Design: Matthew Bartlett, Wellington
Printer: Ligare, Auckland

All rights reserved. No part of this publication may be reproduced, stored in a retrieval system, transmitted or utilized in any form or any means, electronic, mechanical, photocopying, recording or otherwise, without permission in writing from the author, except within an educational institution, where one chapter or ten percent, whichever is the lesser, may be copied for educational purposes only, and except in the case of brief quotation used within critical articles and reviews.

CONTENTS

PART 3: SOME PRAGMATICS FOR PRACTICE

PART 6: EXTENDING ETHICS:THE FUTURE IS ALREADY AT HAND

In the interests of simplicity, throughout the text references to the NZAC *Code of Ethics* will follow a bracketed number format.

ACKNOWLEDGEMENTS

We gratefully acknowledge colleagues who have provided leadership in counselling ethics in New Zealand, particularly within the New Zealand Association of Counsellors, its Executive, and its National Ethics Committee; the contributors to this book who have generously shared their experiences and knowledge; Jenny Snowdon, for editorial assistance at the final stages of the preparation of the text; and the Faculty of Education Research Committee, University of Waikato. We also acknowledge Liz Price for the cover concept.

PART 1

SITUATING COUNSELLING ETHICS IN AOTEAROA NEW ZEALAND

1.1
ETHICS AS EVERYDAY PRACTICE

Kathie Crocket

Ethics comes to life on a daily basis, moment by moment, in the actions we take as counsellors in our counselling practices. Ethical questions are present in every client meeting, in our publicity leaflets, in funding applications, in records of our client work, as we engage in supervision, as we consider ongoing professional education, as we speak formally with colleagues in our own and other professions, or as we speak informally with our colleagues over coffee. The focus of this book is the ethics of everyday counselling practice.

On one hand the ethics of everyday practice tends to take the form of a concern, almost legal in character, amongst practitioners to reduce potential liabilities in order to avoid complaint or prosecution. This approach to ethical relationship is shaped by the responsibilities of a "contractual obligation" (Bauman, 1998), emphasising *rules* of ethical conduct. The assumption that rules can be defined, and thus risk managed, is a familiar feature of neo-liberal societies. As a guide for practitioners, this book actively traverses and engages with this territory. In particular, it interacts with the *Code of Ethics* of the New Zealand Association of Counsellors (NZAC) (2002). It engages with the Code's principles and values, and rules and guidelines of ethical conduct, from the perspective of reducing potential liabilities. But codes of ethics do not always give a clear signal of what the ethical obligations of a particular situation might be. A code is an attempt to deal with ethically problematic situations but it can never be comprehensive, nor anticipate every event that might occur. In everyday practice practitioners are faced with ambiguity and contradictions, and competing ethical values may make the way forward unclear. Engaging with questions produced by ambiguity and contradiction in ethical practice is also a central purpose of this text.

Questions of ambiguity and contradiction take us to a second form of ethics as everyday practice. Beyond an interest in reducing liabilities or a concern for professional and personal safety, counsellors hold a genuine concern to treat people morally, to be in ethical relation with clients and others. Questions of how to be in ethical relation take us into recognising and holding the tension of competing ethical principles and values, and also into philosophical questions about the nature of ethical relationship. In Bauman's words, this expression of ethics is "*to take responsibility for one's responsibility*" (1998). In this task of taking responsibility for one's responsibility, the concerns of moral philosophy echo backwards and forwards into the ethics of the everyday in counselling practice. This echo can be heard in questions of the relationship between the self and the other; of the moral value of recognising the other as different; of how to enact responsibility to the other; and of how to take account of power. For professionals engaging in the practical implications of these questions, suggested Hugman (2005), more recent developments in social thought – such as feminism, ecology, postmodernism – offer language and concepts to promote the possibility of congruence between ethics and practice. Associated with these developments in social thought are a range of approaches to ethics –such as an ethics of care (Gilligan, 1982; Sevenhuijsen, 2003); of emotion and compassion (Nussbaum, 2009); of risk (Welch, 1990); Levinas' (1989) and Bauman's (2000) interest in the face of the Other; and Foucault's (1988) care of the self. These contributions take us directly to questions of moral philosophy that are lived out in the actions practitioners both take, and refrain from taking, in professional practice.

> Capacities such as compassion, attentiveness, discernment, caring, and kindness are integral to the way wise moral agents balance diverse and sometimes competing moral considerations. (Beauchamp & Childress, 2009, p. 22)

Seen in this way, the practice of ethics is an ongoing project.

In the simplest terms, this project is about enacting a commitment to doing good in situations and practices where there is the potential for good or for harm in the context of the responsibilities of professional relationship. The NZAC *Code of Ethics* says: "Counselling involves the formation of professional relationships based on ethical values and principles" (2).

In forming professional relationships in counselling, counsellors take up responsibilities. These responsibilities are to our clients (as people in networks of relational connection), to ourselves, and to the communities of which they are part and we are part. These communities include our agencies, our profession, and the wider communities in which we practise and in which we and our clients live. Thus, while we might most often meet with clients in the privacy of a counselling room, our actions also have a public effect, for our practice takes place in the context of clients' lives, of a profession and of our communities, local and global.

Learning and applying sensitivity for ethical questions that arise in our practice is no less important than learning and applying any other counselling skill or attitude. Continuing to develop and hone our ethical sensitivities is no less important than any other aspect of our ongoing professional development.

Ethical sensitivity involves, first of all, understanding that ethics are woven, moment by moment, into our counselling practices, and so cultivating an attitude of ethical-mindedness. If both ethics and therapy are about power in relationships, as Loewenthal and Snell (2001) argued, "ethics as practice is not in any way separate from psychotherapy" (p. 23). From this perspective, we can attune ourselves to the possible nuances of our own and others' actions, and have an ear for the kinds of relational ethics that are unfolding as we work with others, and that require us to make ongoing professional judgements.

Practice: Thinking about values as we select our responses

Let's think for a moment about the example of a new client telling us that they had seen the counsellor down the street, who they found not very effective. In selecting how to respond we have before us the potential for harm at the same time as our intention is to do good. Different theoretical positions will offer us different ways of interpreting what the client might mean by their comment about the other counsellor, and then deciding how we might respond. For example, some theoretical positions might understand the client's action as representing avoidance or resistance, particularly if we hold this counsellor in high regard; while other theoretical positions might align with a discourse of clients' rights. Whatever our theoretical position, there is a call for us to respond in ethical relation. In responding we carry responsibilities to a new client, to colleagues, to the profession, and to the wider community. There is no neutral position to take. Any response, or non-response, speaks to the relational ethics of counselling practice: this is ethics in action.

I invite you to pause for a moment and think about how you might respond in this situation, where a client speaks about disappointment with services offered by a counsellor down the road:

- What questions might you ask yourself as you think about the situation?
- What questions do you imagine other counsellors in your community might ask?
- What do you notice about the ethical values that your responses and questions might express?

The NZAC *Code of Ethics* (NZAC, 2002) lists these as the six core values of counselling:

1. Respect for human dignity;
2. Partnership;
3. Autonomy;
4. Responsible caring;
5. Personal integrity;
6. Social justice.

In what ways do you see the responses you might have made as embracing these values? Are there other possible actions that might also demonstrate these values? Are there other values you would wish to embrace as you respond, values that are shared with others in your community, or that come out of your particular history? We hope that you will keep these kinds of questions and reflections alive as you continue reading the book.

ETHICS IN PRACTICE: ETHICAL SENSITIVITY

Central to a practice of ethics is the development of sensitivity to "the moral dimensions of counseling" (Welfel, 2006, p. 23). Counsellors might develop and refine this sensitivity by paying attention to what they notice in their practice, and then further exploring what they have noticed. An example follows, to show the working out of ethical sensitivities in everyday practice.

Ethical sensitivity: Noticing what we notice

Jeremy is a relationship counsellor working with Sarah and Peter, in his private practice. Sarah and Peter come to counselling saying that they want to "improve communication" between them. When Jeremy asks them how they are hoping things will be different in their relationship when communication is improved, both Sarah and Peter speak in terms of Sarah "stopping her nagging." They speak of Sarah's "constant nagging" and Peter says that Sarah is "just like her mother," that both women have nagged all their lives. Sarah does not dispute Peter's descriptions.

Listening with ethical sensitivity, Jeremy notices that while Sarah and Peter's hopes were for improved communication between them, the descriptions they have been offering locate the difficulty in one person in the couple, in Sarah and her "constant nagging." These kinds of descriptions that identify one person as responsible for relationship difficulties are not unfamiliar to Jeremy as a relationship counsellor: he knows this is a common way for people to understand the difficulties they encounter as a couple. As well, Jeremy's experience is that, despite the advances that feminism has brought, it is not unusual for a woman partner to be held responsible for difficulties: nagging is a description that tends to be applied to women, rather than to men.

Jeremy's noticing here is linked with both professional and personal values. As a young undergraduate psychology student in the 1970s, he was introduced to the work by Broverman, Broverman, Clarkson, Rosencrantz and Vogel (1970), who argued that adjustment to stereotypical sex roles did not serve the mental health of men or women. Their study suggested that mental health professionals considered that a typical "healthy woman" is more submissive, less adventurous, more easily influenced, less competitive, more emotional, and less objective than a hypothetical healthy man or adult (gender unspecified). Then, as a social worker in the 1980s, he found the Just Therapy team's explorations of gender and culture helpful, and had taken to heart their suggestion that therapy that does not "seek out the gender context and meaning associated with it will often entrench the problem further" (Waldegrave, 1990, p. 29). Moving into counselling in the 1990s, Jeremy continued to weave into his practice the knowledges offered by feminist writers and practitioners. "Knowledge and practice are not neutral, and feminists must maintain vigilant attention to assuring that their practices do not subtly reinforce the very practices that they have attempted to eradicate, reform, or transform" (Enns, 1993, p. 64). As a male counsellor working mainly with couples, Jeremy continues to take seriously his responsibility for a socially just practice. He pays careful attention to the NZAC *Code of Ethics*, identifying the core values as involving particular responsibilities for ethical sensitivity. In this situation these responsibilities include considering how relationship difficulties are described and understood. Jeremy does not want to reproduce gender, or other, injustice in his practice.

Thinking in terms of these kinds of ethical sensitivities, Jeremy identifies an in-the-moment ethical question in his practice: will he use the words and concepts Peter and Sarah are using to describe and understand the difficulties they are experiencing in their relationship? He asks himself about potential for harm. What harm might be done by continuing to use these words and concepts? He believes that, as a male counsellor, his use of the words would likely have the effect of shoring up male privilege. However, at these early stages of building a therapeutic relationship, he is aware of some potential for harm in not using the language Sarah and Peter have used. If he moves too quickly in making other ideas and words available, they might experience him as not listening to their experience, and therefore as not joining them in the partnership of counselling.

Jeremy takes into account the responsibilities he has as a counsellor to promote the safety and well-being of (4.5), and increase the range of choices and opportunities for (4.6), the couple who are his clients. These are the two ethical principles he identifies as important here.

In this example, Jeremy noticed the in-the-moment ethical question that arose for him in the everyday matter of deciding what words he would use. He then set the question that he noticed in the context of this meeting as relationship therapy, in the wider professional culture, and in the personal and professional values he brings to his practice. Each of these contexts offered him opportunity to further notice and identify the complexity of the ethical question. Of significance here is Jeremy's work in *noticing*, and going on to *contextualise*, the ethical questions arising in his ordinary daily practice. These questions arise out of the context of Jeremy's own life and professional commitments, and in the context of a particular culture. What might Jeremy notice if, as a New Zealand-born Chinese person, he was to work with a couple recently arrived from Taiwan, for example? Or if Jeremy, a gay man, were to learn that the problem had arisen since Peter's brother had told Sarah and Peter he was leaving his marriage for a same-sex relationship?

The development of ethical sensitivities takes places within the cultural contexts of our communities, for these communities, and our relationships in them, shape our professional practices. We hope that your engagement with the various sections of this book will help you hone sensitivities for the ethical questions of your own counselling practice. This example highlights a particular understanding of ethics that suggests that our ethical responsibilities cannot be defined in advance of a particular situation and interaction, but require in-the-moment ethical sensitivities and responsiveness.

ABOUT THIS BOOK

This book aims to locate the ethics of practice in the context of counselling in Aotearoa New Zealand. While the NZAC *Code of Ethics* shares some central values with other professional codes, in New Zealand and elsewhere, it espouses values unique to counselling, and to counselling in New Zealand. In particular the NZAC *Code of Ethics* refers in its introduction to the Treaty of Waitangi, and invokes partnership, in a purposeful echo (see Winslade, 2002) of the principles of the Treaty. In focusing on ethics in practice, and locating this practice in our local Aotearoa New Zealand context, the book's central purpose is to support the ongoing learning and practice of ethical sensitivity and responsibility. We believe that sensitivity to the ethical values and principles that we enact as practitioners is at the centre of the practice of counselling, whatever our chosen practice orientation.

A feature of this book is its many authors. Many local practitioners have joined in offering both reflections on and guidelines for ethical practice. In this way the book brings together the knowledges and resources of many communities of practice. The authors of the various contributions in this book offer examples from the local context, interweaving these with literature from international perspectives. Each of these practitioners has taken a focus on a particular area of interest and expertise, drawing on practice wisdom and current literature. They all bring experience in particular practice contexts, as well as leadership in aspects of professional ethics. The authors of the different sections in this book write in a range of styles. They also write from a range of theoretical perspectives, each in their preferred way expressing the shared values of the profession. We acknowledge and thank them for their contributions to our field, and particularly to this book and the practice of those who read it.

Our hope in bringing together the ideas of this wide range of authors is that this book will support counsellors and counselling communities as we take seriously our responsibilities to develop ethical sensitivity, including the steps of recognition, thoughtfulness and action. Such sensitivity recognises that each of us, as members of our wider communities, creates the ethos of counselling practice moment-by-moment.

Part One offers a general orientation to ethics in practice. This orientation encourages us to think about both the wider vision and values of our practice, and the particularities of an Aotearoa context.

Part Two considers the responsibilities of presenting ourselves as professionals and has sections on advertising, professional disclosure statements, private practice settings, working beyond agency walls, soliciting clients, seeking client testimonials, and research and publication.

The pragmatics of practice are the focus of Part Three. Sections include notes about notes, confidentiality for school counsellors, even-handedness in relationship counselling, multiple relationships, managing complex relationships in pastoral and church-based counselling, complex relationships in LGBTI communities, working within the scope of our competence, unbearable affect, touch in counselling, when a client dies, communicating with other professionals, online practices, electronic recording of counselling conversations, ethical responsibility towards others in a client's life, and imminent threat of serious harm.

In Part Four the emphasis is on the intersection of ethics and the law. This part should be read alongside Ludbrook's (2003) New Zealand volume.

There are times when things go wrong, through oversight, failure to notice, misjudgement, or even when we have intended to take reasonable steps to protect clients from harm. Part Five has as its focus those times when the ethics of our practice come under question.

The book concludes with Part Six, when once again the ethics of our counselling practice are situated in the context of our values and responsibilities as professionals and as persons in the world.

> For the ethical world, however, ambivalence and uncertainty are its daily bread and butter and cannot be stamped out without destroying the moral substance of responsibility, the foundation on which that world rests. (Bauman, 2000, p. 10)

Acknowledgement

I acknowledge the contribution of Hamish Crocket, whose scholarship in ethics in sport has shaped my thinking about ethics in counselling.

1.2
TE TIRITI AND ETHICS AS DIALOGUE: A UNIQUE CALL TO PARTNERSHIP?

Joy Te Wiata and Alastair Crocket,
with reflections from Vi Woolf and Carl Mika

This next section calls readers to enter a space where difference is given voice. It is a unique difference, specific to Aotearoa New Zealand. The voices that you are called to hear are Joy and Alastair as they kōrero their respective relationships to the Treaty of Waitangi and its import for ethics in practice. In this piece, they make visible the struggle to come together towards dialogue. As editors, we value this transparency for it sets the tone for the ways in which counsellors might also struggle to open spaces to speak into difference in our own practices. Although it cannot be known in advance where such kōrero will lead, we find hope in the ways in which Joy and Alastair show themselves as willing to be changed in dialogue, thus opening space for difference.

Brief reflections on Joy's and Alastair's kōrero are offered by Vi Woolf, and then Carl Mika. Their reflections give further voice to difference, highlighting the importance of opening spaces for multiple perspectives in dialogue about difference and partnership.

This section considers two questions in particular:

- How do we see the connections between the Treaty of Waitangi/ te Tiriti o Waitangi and the NZAC *Code of Ethics*?
- How might we draw from the Treaty's/te Tiriti's guidance to shape ethical counselling practice?

Alastair begins: I have come to understand the Treaty documents as the record of an agreement between peoples that laid the foundation for Aotearoa New Zealand as a nation. From these agreements, the Treaty today is situated in a broader context, supporting aspirations about the kind of political, social and personal relationships that we might achieve. In this way there is direct relevance to counselling, demonstrated by references to the Treaty in the NZAC *Code of Ethics*. The introduction states:

> Counsellors shall seek to be informed about the meaning and implications of the Treaty of Waitangi for their work. They shall understand the principles of protection, participation and partnership with Maori.

Partnership is also a Core Value, and the third of the Ethical Principles states that "counsellors shall [a]ctively support the principles embodied in the Treaty of Waitangi" (4.3). I believe that together these statements centre the Treaty in the Code. They suggest that counsellors should understand the Treaty and the principles as part of ethical practice in Aotearoa New Zealand.

Because of the particular emphasis the Code gives to partnership as a Core Value of counselling, perhaps we might specifically consider partnership in this discussion?

Joy responds: As I consider the Treaty of Waitangi and ethical practice, it is with an acknowledgement that the current ideas I hold of the Treaty and its intent are partial. As a Māori practitioner in Aotearoa New Zealand, in the Pākehā-dominated discipline of counselling, it is my understanding that historically, where Treaty considerations have informed the *Code of Ethics*, reference has understandably been to the English version of the Treaty.

However, as work continues in understanding te Tiriti, the original document in te reo Māori, fundamental differences between the two versions continue to mount. Therefore, ideas and ethical considerations generated from partial understandings of the document must be constantly available for review and revision.

I take up your comment about viewing te Tiriti as "supporting aspirations about the kind of political, social and personal relationships that we might achieve." I would take that further to have us consider that te Tiriti opens space for people to consider and embrace multiple strands of relationship that produce the kinds of political, social, personal and therapeutic relationships that are unique to Aotearoa New Zealand.

One of the challenges presented when considering the Treaty and the *Code of Ethics* is producing a consensus of understanding in regard to basic Treaty principles. Since tino rangatiratanga was never ceded by Iwi, I understand te Tiriti as an agreement between sovereign nations that was initially instigated so that each sovereign nation would take responsibility for the care and governance of their own. So taking up the notion of partnership, do we assume that practitioners hold a consensus of understanding of the nature of that partnership? For Māori and Pākehā to move forward together, the Treaty partnership needs to be acknowledged and embraced as a partnership of sovereigns. It may be agreed that partnership infers equality, but for some this may equate with 'sameness'. The challenge is to embrace the richness of diversity as well as to celebrate shared places of understanding.

Alastair: Joy, your comment that our understandings of the Treaty/te Tiriti are partial offers me the opportunity to reflect and notice how easily I can still slip into references, such as "the Treaty," which give support to Pākehā thinking and values more than to Māori thinking and values. In response to your kōrero, I am reflecting that I am still strongly influenced by texts written in English. There is a risk that actions from this position marginalise Māori understandings about te Tiriti.

With these points in mind, I offer these further thoughts more tentatively. I have suggested that partnership translates well as a Treaty principle when I consider collegial relationships in an agency or between an agency and a kindred Māori agency or roopu (Crocket, 2009). However, in terms of counsellor–client relationships I have found it helpful to think about the *spirit of partnership*, which was a usage promoted by the Royal Commission on Social Policy (1988) when it was charged with identifying Treaty principles. Nonetheless, I want to keep open to considering how these ideas may be reshaped in dialogue with Māori understandings about partnership, and I acknowledge the importance of your call for Pākehā/Tauiwi[1] acceptance of tino rangatiratanga and the consequent effects of this acceptance on our practice.

These considerations lead me to ask you, Joy, if you would think that it is important to acknowledge the years of Treaty/Tiriti work with its pains and achievements?

1 A Māori term for "other people". This is a way of referring to people of other-than-Māori descent.

Joy: I agree it is critical we remember the whakapapa of the journey towards redressing some of the injustices and pain produced by colonising practices. Te Tiriti continues to offer us a way forward in this respect. My concern as a practitioner is that energy is often expended in trying to find a way forward together that can be compromising of both Tiriti partners, resulting in diluted outcomes. Alternatively, one partner may experience themselves as bending over backwards for the other, making sweeping changes that ultimately impair the relationships they are seeking to advance and enhance. Either way, all are at risk of not benefiting from the richness that diversity can offer.

Alastair: When I hear you speak of diversity, I think of the Treaty as also inviting personal consideration of the spectrum of identities and relationships that make up Aotearoa New Zealand. I feel called to identify as Pākehā and in this I acknowledge that my predecessors were involved in the settlement of land, which may have been unfairly purchased from Māori, and that one effect of that purchase was that the people in the area had less access to resources they needed for their preferred way of life. I intend this identification to contribute to acknowledgment of the painful effects of colonisation and to commitment to addressing these effects professionally, socially and politically. At the same time I acknowledge that a binary of Māori/Pākehā may contribute to feelings of marginalisation for those who do not or cannot take up either identity. However, for me, my identification as Pākehā is a first step towards partnership relationships.

As a Pākehā counsellor this means that I consider both the colonial history and my contribution to addressing its consequences. I know that I am identified by those I work with as a member of the dominant culture of Aotearoa. Through taking up ideas inherent in a spirit of partnership, I hope to work in ways that do not engage in further exercises of colonisation.

Joy: Some Pākehā practitioners have also shared with me stories of pain stemming from their experiences of learning to work cross-culturally during the 1980s. They found their endeavours to honour Māori in their work made them vulnerable to the charge of co-opting Māori language and knowledges and thus participating in the further colonising of Māori. Over time, they report a progression in the move from participating in colonising practices, which produce Māori as subjugated subjects, towards practices that open space to negotiate meaning as a way forward, to produce mutually honouring relationships between Māori and Pākehā

(Te Wiata, 2006). Arguably this has been made more possible by a growing confidence in Pākehā identity possibilities. Though there is much uncharted territory in the ongoing story of Pākehā identity construction, there is an identification by some practitioners that Māori cultural ideas, practices, and values have contributed to their accounts of identity.

Holding this understanding of the unique identities produced in this land, and considering the complexities of partnership relationships, I believe Māori values can offer both Māori and Pākehā a way to experience relationship and to practice in ways that some more widely accepted Western psychological practices may not offer. Aotearoa New Zealand practitioners are delightfully positioned to be frontrunners in generating practices that draw directly from Māori cultural wisdoms and Māori clinical practice to produce ethical practice in all communities. Ongoing attention to practices of remembering, honouring and acknowledgement would be required to support this way forward. To me this is the spirit of partnership.

The following is an example of how Māori values can shape practice. Māori cultural precepts, based on intentionally seeking, acknowledging and declaring our connectedness, offer a foundation for approaching relationships as Treaty partners: inter-agency, collegial, client–counsellor therapeutic intervention. They do this by inviting us to trace our ancestry, our whakapapa, until we find a link between the 'other' and ourselves. Between Māori this is most often a genealogical link. At other times it may be a significant historical event that creates the link. Importantly, we recognise each other as whānau/kin and, in its broadest sense for Māori, there is no-one who exists beyond kinship links. The same process is extended to manuhiri, or visitors, and for the purpose of the event or the work to be done, the manuhiri become whānau. Interwoven in the connecting process is the notion of shared rights and responsibility. Whether colleague, therapist or client, each takes up their responsibility as kin or partners in the project to ensure its success. Thus, by purposefully seeking strands of relationship and honouring those relationships, mutual investment in the project is established and enhanced.

These practices introduce a particular complexity in terms of the ethics of overlapping relationships. While Tomm (1993) advocated for the admission of dual relationships in the therapeutic context on the basis of acknowledging "human connectedness" (p. 48), his advocacy stopped short of purposefully seeking connectedness as a way of enhancing professional therapeutic relationship. In contrast, Māori values and practices offer a way forward by purposefully seeking and embracing multiple strands of relationship to produce partnership, thus displacing ideas that might otherwise limit connection and promote separation.

We hear a call to partnership in this nation that is unique to us. We can choose to embrace our geographical isolation, our small population and limited degrees of separation. We can embrace the richness of our cultural heritages, the uniqueness of our Pākehā and Māori identities and the opportunities that we have together as sovereign Treaty partners. We can join our voices together as confident Treaty partners to create best practice in Aotearoa New Zealand, the roots of which are firmly located in our local context.

1.2a Reflection on 'Te Tiriti and ethics as dialogue: A unique call to partnership?' — Vi Woolf

Kia ora to Joy and Alastair and their kōrero.

Joy and Alastair's conversation is one of many kinds of conversation that counsellors might have about te Tiriti and counselling ethics. Other conversations might have the flavours of "back home," of people yarning together in local communities. Some conversations might use language that is more organic, local and everyday. Some conversations might involve just one Treaty partner – iwi, for example, talking about common experiences. What is important is that understandings of partnership continue to grow and develop.

1.2b A second reflection on 'Te Tiriti and ethics as dialogue: A unique call to partnership?' — Carl Mika

As I read the reflections on partnership and counselling, I would also urge the consideration of other more nebulous questions. In supporting these questions to emerge, one could begin by provocatively asserting that Māori are not only physical entities but also carry with them their ancestors (quite alongside their ancestry), the emotional and spiritual layering provided by their whenua, the unseen and unperceivable, indeterminate world, and so on. Indeed, these are givens in much Māori scholarship (Pere, 1982; Royal, 2003, 2009); however, there is a call for their active role to be explored in counselling, if Māori are to have any say in how the practice of counselling occurs. The questions following from such a declaration then need to be ongoing rather than terminal. For instance, we might start with: how important is the *place* in which counselling occurs? Does counselling need to acknowledge *place*, and should it occur in a whakapapa-derived *place*?

Even more uncomfortably, there is reason now to call into question how the very discipline of counselling, in its necessary identification of the Māori client as an *Other* entity, affects those subtle, but real, layers that Māori bring with them into the arena of problem/resolution. Counselling by its very nature exists because a dilemma is intended as a focus. Does that very intention construct the Māori client's responses narrowly, thereby influencing the deeper ontological spheres that come with the spirit, mentality and emotion? How does the practice and language of counselling, in enacting this search for a resolution, impact on the very body of the Māori client? The freedom to ask these and other sorts of questions – without having to produce solutions – necessarily raises the anxiety levels of not only counsellors but also other professionals, who may think of their practices as largely disembodied activities. If anything, any partnership derived from Treaty expectations encourages the continual posing of questions that seek to both critique and construct possible other forms of practice.

1.3
CULTURE IS ALWAYS PRESENT: A CONVERSATION ABOUT ETHICS

Margaret Agee, Kathie Crocket, Carol Fatialofa, Kaaren Frater-Mathieson, Hyeeun Kim, Candy Vong and Vi Woolf

"There isn't any daylight between culture and ethics," one of us comments. Across our different perspectives we nod in agreement. Coming together as a collegial community, we seven meet together on a winter's evening, sharing food, and sharing ideas and experiences about the interrelationship of culture and ethics. Though some already know each other well and others know few present, our common purpose draws us together. So what is it about this idea, that there is no daylight between culture and ethics, that it resonates with each of us?

All of us, counsellors and clients, are shaped by the cultures in which we have grown up, in which we live our lives, and in which we encounter one another – and by the histories of those cultures and the relationships between them. At the same time, the ways in which clients and counsellors encounter one another in therapeutic relationships are shaped by personal and professional ethics, and by relations of power. For example, how counsellors "promote the safety and well-being of individuals, families, communities, whanau, hapu and iwi" (NZAC, 2002, 4.5) depends upon the cultural understandings of safety and well-being associated with particular cultural contexts, and the ways in which people are positioned within those contexts. In one cultural setting a career counsellor assisting a mother into employment, might also think in terms of the wider family situation that constrains the possibilities available to the mother. Thus, Carol suggests, having learned from a mother of her concerns for her adolescent children if she returns to work, a counsellor might also network with the justice system and with school counsellors. In working with the whole family, and developing a network of support, a counsellor acts on the basis that the well-being of a mother, her direct client, is inevitably tied up with the well-being of her children. Carol later speaks in terms of two accountabilities, to both an "ethical base" and a "cultural base." Her task, she suggests, is to keep ethics and culture in dialogue with each other.

Immediately illuminating diversity, Candy reports her experience of a family meeting that included a child, parents and other relatives. The meeting had been called to discuss the child's difficulties. However, in this cultural context, a meeting with the wider family had not been appropriate because of the shame of disclosure, and the ongoing effects for the family of losing face amongst the wider family. While one cultural context calls for beginning counselling by reaching out to family, another calls for more bounded participation.

Thus we agree that the pathways towards the safety and well-being of individuals, families, communities, whānau, hapū and iwi are not clearly signposted, but require some particular skills in map reading, and ongoing consultation with other travellers, most particularly clients, along the way. A counsellor's ethical map-reading is made even more complex by the shifting landscapes of cultural identification and practice (see Abu-Lughod, 2006; Culbertson & Agee, 2007, for example). If we do not recognise the shifting nature of these landscapes, there is a risk of making assumptions about particular cultural groups or cultural differences.

A story from Hyeeun illustrates this cultural complexity:

> Only two or three years after my migration I was still a very Korean girl, a 'good girl'. There was also the influence of my family culture: my father was a minister, my mother was a teacher, so I was the 'good girl' who listened to authority ... So when I disagreed with a social worker about uplifting a child from her family, all I could do was to say, "Oh, I don't think that is right."
>
> Later in my career, in a similar situation, I had the support of my agency and of training, and I looked at the client and I *had* to do something as a professional. Then I had my voice. I could choose to be an advocate and an educator: this was a New Zealand context and I had a responsibility for the well-being of my client and their family.
>
> At the same time I do not think it is ethical to push a person against their own preference. And of course, any preference they express is also a product of their cultural context and experiences. We need to take this into account in thinking about what actions will promote safety and well-being for them.

> Another counsellor from a similar cultural background might have responded differently in either of these situations, because of different life experiences. When I think about these different client situations, in some ways I think I am not 'Korean' anymore. I am a Korean but some parts of me are not Korean anymore, because I have been here in New Zealand long enough, or perhaps too long.

Hyeeun's story makes many important points in terms of ethical practice. Firstly there is the caution against making assumptions based on ethnicity or appearance: what does it mean to be Korean and live in New Zealand? Or what might it mean to have been born of New Zealand parents living Japan, and to return to New Zealand as a young adult? Or to identify as Māori and have blonde hair and blue eyes? There are dangers in over-generalising, in the limiting ideas of singular belongings and identifications, and in making assumptions based on incomplete knowledge. As Candy notes: "Someone says, 'Oh, he is Chinese,' but if he comes from mainland China, it's really different from someone who comes from Hong Kong or Taiwan." Candy also notes the challenges for a counsellor negotiating between a family and agencies when "the same Chinese family has different members with different levels of acculturation to New Zealand culture." Given the potential for misunderstanding and conflict, actions to increase the range of choices and opportunities available to individual family members might not be congruent with the safety and well-being of the family as a unit, or of particular family members.

Acting with care and respect for individual differences and the diversity of human experience (4.1) requires that we both recognise cultural difference and work to understand the possible variations in the significance of those differences, both *between* cultures and *within* cultures.

Cultural identity is complex: as Carol comments, "Our experience of our own culture may be different from the person sitting next to us." Cultural theorist Benhabib (2002) made a similar point: "To the participants and the actors, their culture presents itself as a set of competing as well as cohering accounts" (p. 103). Differences and similarities are both present within any cultural group, and even within a family, as Candy points out. While noting that "as part of the way that people give meaning to their world, culture will always be inescapable" (p. 15), Phillips (2007) also suggested that "culture talk" tends to obscure many variations within cultures (p. 133). Anthropologist Abu-Lughod (2006) wrote about the implications of these ideas for everyday living.

> The particulars [of people's lives] suggest that others live as we perceive ourselves living, not as robots programmed with "cultural" rules, but as people going through life agonizing over decisions, making mistakes, trying to make themselves look good, enduring tragedies and personal losses, enjoying others, and finding moments of happiness. (p. 164)

Thus when we meet people in our counselling rooms, we might always assume that culture has a shaping effect on how they are enduring a tragedy, for example, but we cannot assume that culture can be thought of as singular or definitive of that person's experience. This is the point that Hyeeun and Carol are making: that we must listen to preferences people express, within the contexts of their lives and relationships, rather than assume that behaviour will conform to a predetermined cultural model about which we have learned. Practitioners are thus called into complex navigation as we endeavour to act with care and respect for difference. This brings us to the question of what we do when faced with ethical challenges in working in an unfamiliar cultural situation, a second point that Hyeeun's story raises for us.

While Hyeeun tells of finding a voice to advocate and educate, counsellors from the dominant culture have a further responsibility to position ourselves to learn when we do not have access to particular ethno-cultural knowledge. At the least, we practitioners might acknowledge the ethno-cultural expertise that our clients bring to counselling. Hyeeun later pointed to her responsibilities as a Korean counsellor to consult with Māori and Pasifika clients about their particular cultural interpretations. The responsibility to consult clients or others who might offer cultural guidance is shared by all practitioners. Our relational responsibility is maybe to know that we do not know – to recognise our own areas of cultural ignorance – in order to avoid potential harms arising from what Bell (2008) described as "ignorance (or knowledge) as domination" (p. 864). At the same time, the ethical concern to avoid acting in domination of those who are culturally different does not absolve us from professional responsibility, when, for example, not knowing may be an insufficient response alongside our professional responsibilities for socially just practice. Referring to such responsibilities, Kaaren asks: "How do we work with the elusiveness of power that is embedded and hidden within our institutions?"

As well as consulting between cultures, within-culture consultations can be important in acting with *care and respect* for difference and diversity (5.2). Candy speaks about consulting her colleagues who bring cultural knowledge similar to her own. In a situation where she had noticed unease, she had paused and asked about the possible cultural meanings of a family meeting. Through investigating and sharing culture-specific knowledge, Candy was strengthened in her concern and supported in advocating for practices that might enhance the safety and well-being of the family. But as our conversation keeps noticing, it might not always be the case that the views of two persons of similar culture are aligned. Writing of therapy and structural difference, Burman (2004) suggested that the task is to "*work with* such differences, rather than portraying them as obstacles to be overcome on the road to some fictional universalised state of complete mutual understanding or relatedness" (pp. 293–294). Monk, Winslade and Sinclair (2008) wrote of a "vision" of counselling that "welcome[s] people and offer[s] them hospitality on the very basis of their difference" (p. 461).

As our conversation draws to an end, Vi comments on the priority the NZAC *Code of Ethics* gives to partnership, and continues:

> We are actually in partnership now in this group. We are talking about our cultural base, which widens out the idea of partnership a great deal more.

Vi expresses concern and hope that, when counselling becomes a registered profession, we will find ways to maintain and build on the progress made within NZAC to honour partnership.

From our different experiences and perspectives, as we have worked with differences, we seem to have come to agree on some general principles to shape our thinking about ethics and culture. We have spoken of culture and difference as fluid and complex. We have noticed the slipperiness, and incompleteness, of cultural identifiers. We have each, and differently, noticed our knowing and our not knowing. We have noticed that difference can call us into the possibility of dialogue, but that speaking positions might not be equally available to all. Our shared hope is for ongoing dialogue at the intersections of ethics and culture.

1.4 SITUATING ETHICAL PRACTICE IN PHILOSOPHICAL STORYLINES

Sue Cornforth and Kathie Crocket

While the story of ethics is as old as and perhaps older than the Hippocratic Oath, contemporary ethical codes also emerge out of commitments to social justice and a desire to form inclusive societies. Any discussion of justice involves a consideration of power – political, social and economic – and inclusion involves reconsideration of the effects of power, both within and beyond counselling rooms and centres. Shaped by discourses of race, culture, gender, ability, sexual orientation and so on, counselling practice is embedded within relationships of power, and the ways these relationships of power work out in people's lives. Counsellors are constantly brought face to face with the individual effects of complex processes of minoritisation (Chantler, 2005) that exclude many clients from full participation in society. While, day-to-day, counsellors may think of themselves as responding on a practical level to the effects of these complex processes, this responding is shaped by a series of philosophical and historical storylines. This section briefly traces some of these interweaving storylines, which shape how we proceed in our professional practice. While these storylines interweave in shaping ethical thinking and practice, the account we offer here highlights separate threads in turn. We do this to show how each storyline carries within it particular conceptual tools that help make sense of the actions we think of as ethics.

THE STORYLINE OF THE SOCIAL CONTRACT

One longstanding sociopolitical challenge is found in the question of how a diverse group of people joins together to form a society. This is a problem that troubled early philosophers such as Hobbes (1651), Locke (1690) and Rousseau (1762). The problem is often discussed in relation to the "social contract" (Rousseau), and framed in terms of those rights and responsibilities people accord to each other, or give up, in order to live harmoniously together. Using this storyline, professional codes might be seen as formal statements of each profession's social contract, both between that profession and the wider society, and between members of the profession. Counselling, however, is caught up in regimes and techniques of power, with the potential for both liberatory and oppressive effects (Fairclough, 1992). Thus, it can be argued that in prioritising the well-being of clients, counsellors should understand the regimes and techniques of power in which counselling is caught up. Such understanding, Waldegrave (1990) suggested, would lead counsellors to refuse to neutralise in the counselling room what they learn there about suffering, particularly that produced through minoritisation and injustice. Rather, counsellors' responsibility, in terms of the social contract, is to speak into the domains of social policy and practice. A further responsibility in terms of service to the community is to act as conduits or brokers of services, as "intermediaries between systems (educational, healthcare, employment) and individuals" (American Counseling Association, 2005, as cited in Paredes et al., 2008, p. 156), thus making systems more accessible to those who need their services. These responsibilities can be seen in the NZAC *Code of Ethics*, for example, "counsellors should be committed to the equitable provision of counselling services to all individuals and social groups" (5.2g); "counsellors shall promote social justice through advocacy and empowerment (5.2.h); "counsellors are encouraged to contribute to policy direction" (8.2.d); and "counsellors shall inform clients, where relevant, of the availability of government funding for counselling services" (5.5e).

The social contract also involves a storyline of the particular kind of relationship that is produced between client and counsellor: this is a value-laden relationship. As Small (2008) noted in reference to teaching: "people expect professions to go beyond what is strictly required by any contractual setting in terms of personal commitment. They also expect them to observe higher standards of conduct than other occupations" (p. 60). In counselling this has been spoken of as a covenantal relationship

(Axten, 2004; Doherty, 1995). Based on a duty of care, it involves a "commitment to pursue the good of others in a context of gift, fidelity and trust" (Axten, 2004, p. 105). Current interest in professional ethics and the development, and revision, of ethical codes over the last few decades (Small, 2008), can be seen as an attempt to formalise this "covenantal" relationship and to develop a storyline that takes it beyond mere contractual arrangements into the realm of the moral and the sacred. The covenantal relationship interweaves the storylines of (priestly) pastoral care and secular counselling. The counselling credo emerges from the value-laden nature of this covenantal relationship and is expressed in the core values prioritised in codes of ethics. In the playing out of the covenantal relationship, the caring professions are united around the core value of doing no harm.

CHANGING STORYLINES ABOUT AVOIDING HARM

Considerations of harm are particularly relevant at this time, as the profession of counselling in New Zealand seeks to place itself amongst the health professions registered under the terms of the Health Practitioners Competence Assurance Act (2003). In order to achieve registration, a professional group has to prove that "there is a risk of harm from the practice of the profession" (http://www.moh.govt.nz/hpca). In response to this requirement, the counselling profession in New Zealand has attempted to name and describe the potential for harm in the practice of counselling. It is perhaps not surprising that this description is not straightforward: according to Neiman (2002), a contemporary philosopher, the nature of harm has seldom been put under scrutiny, but is present only in its absence, in being named as something to be avoided. Neiman suggested this avoidance has left a legacy of indecisiveness in response to ethical problems.

Harm challenges our place in the world and how we make meaning. Neiman (2002) traced two impactful events in Euro-western history, the 1755 Lisbon earthquake and the Nazi Holocaust, that each overturned the then dominant story about avoidance of harm. Employing the concept of evil, Neiman posited that the terrible destruction of the Lisbon earthquake destroyed "man's faith in God" to protect the world from evil; while the Holocaust, and the visible presence of harm and evil, destroyed "man's faith in man." She made these claims in reference to the storylines available to make sense of such world-shattering events: that faith protects from harm, or that reason can be used to avoid harm. According to her account, the philosopher Kant is said to have developed his theories as a result of his experiences in Lisbon at the time of the earthquake, which problematised faith in God in the face of such destruction. In response to the question of how an all-powerful God could allow such devastation, he theorised the inherently ethical nature of the "rational man" who, rather than relying on the mystery of prayer as protection from harm, could think his way through difficult situations by obeying certain universal principles that defined ethical conduct and duties. The tradition of faith and the authority of God were, for many, replaced by the storyline of rationality and the authority of science.

The extremely influential Kantian proposition of "the rational man" was, however, severely tested after the revelations of the evils of the Holocaust. How could this same universal, rational man ever again be trusted? Just as the Lisbon earthquake had destabilised the dominant storyline of faith in God as protection against evil, the Holocaust destabilised the dominant storyline of faith in rational man. The shock of witnessing the evidence and aftermath of the Holocaust led various philosophers to declare that we must never let this happen again. In the words of Levinas (1989): "the Other becomes my neighbour precisely through the way the face summons me, calls for me, begs for me, and in so doing recalls my responsibility, and calls me into question" (p. 83). Various alternative storylines of the ethics of the avoidance of harm have emerged in the years since the Holocaust. Each of these has a relational emphasis of some kind. Levinas' (1989) face-to-face ethics of response-ability has been particularly influential; along with Gilligan's (1982) feminist ethics of care, and various indigenous and ecological ethics (see Hugman, 2005).

However, old storylines are persistent and each thread leaves its legacy, offering different positions when it comes to taking ethical action. Taking this history into account, the available dominant ethical stories indicate three interconnecting paths that might be taken by those wanting to avoid harm: prayer, thoughtfulness in relation to certain principles, and emotional and relational responsiveness. Whatever storylines are chosen depends on the interplay of experience and social forces. At stake is the question of how diverse personal realities and social practices shape and form each other. Weaving through these storylines, and, indeed, as Neiman (2002) would argue, as a result of them, are two enduring themes in terms of possible ethical response: does ethical action come out of following rational, universalised rules or does it arise out of a particular and embodied sense of what is right?

STORYLINES OF "OUGHT" AND "IS"

These enduring themes had already appeared at an earlier time in what Hume (1739) called the gap between the "ought" and the "is." In order to maintain a social contract – to acknowledge responsibilities to fellow human beings, and avoid doing harm – there is an important question to be addressed. To what extent are people motivated by adhering to powerful, externally imposed, socially-agreed-upon logical rules – "oughts"? This is sometimes called the deontological approach, and is attributed to Kant. Alternatively, to what extent are people motivated by their own subjective sense of what "is" sensed as right, as advocated by Rousseau and Hume? The dilemma continues to challenge moral thinkers who have framed the problem differently according to their participation in different debates: sometimes in terms of reality and reason (for example, Neiman, 2002), sometimes in terms of relativism and essentialism (Nussbaum, 1992), sometimes in terms of particularism and universalism (see Hugman, 2005).

Some philosophers, such as Neiman (2002), think that the urge to merge the "is" and the "ought" is the origin of all moral thought. Neiman used the stronger, more encompassing concept of evil, rather than harm, to demonstrate its pivotal position in bringing together individuals with their social contexts. She wrote:

> Every time we make the judgment *this [is] ought not to have happened,* we are stepping onto a path that leads straight to the problem of evil [harm] ... At issue are questions about what the structure of the world must be like for us to think and act within it. (p. 5)

If one takes this position, one could say that the desire not to harm impels counsellors to develop both their ethical thinking and their ethical sensitivity, as well as to examine the ways in which their practices inform, and are informed by, wider social contexts. The central value of *doing no harm* is associated with regimes of power that shape the very foundations of NZAC and the way counselling is practised, monitored and accounted for. How counsellors engage with the regimes of power that produce and are produced by counselling requires the development of ethical sensitivities.

INTERWEAVING THE STORYLINES OF ETHICAL SENSITIVITY AND ETHICAL THINKING

In this book we prefer the term *ethical sensitivity* to the more common term *ethical thinking* because we believe it invokes the relational and emotional focus of counselling. We also want to emphasise that people's recognition of, and responses to, ethically challenging situations occur not just cognitively, but in the whole of their being. NZAC attempts to bring together the "is" of subjective experience and the "ought" of professional norms in a two-pronged fashion: by selecting for membership applicants "of good character" (NZAC, 2002, p. 39), that is, people whose ethical sensitivity is considered well developed; and by establishing some core professionally agreed-upon values in the *Code of Ethics*. These core professional values are founded on the work of influential medical ethicists such as Beauchamp and Childress (1994, 2009) who, in 1977, foregrounded the ancient principles of autonomy, beneficence, non-maleficence, fidelity and social justice. These were brought into counselling by Kitchener (1984). Across all the helping professions they form the foundations of ethical thinking, and have been absorbed into professional codes of practice through varying descriptions.

While on the one hand, witnessing of the Holocaust introduced an Other-focused emotionality, at the same time it led to a universal commitment to social justice, expressed in variety of regulatory agreements. While these were to do with the development of medical research ethics in response to publicity about horrific Nazi research experiments during the Third Reich, they have been absorbed into professional codes of practice and are in common parlance across the caring professions. According to Fisher and Anushko (2008), the Nuremberg Code, and subsequent related documents such as the Geneva Convention (1949), the Declaration of Helsinki (1964), and the Belmont Report (1979) in the US, consistently foregrounded three key research principles: autonomy, beneficence and justice (see also Gallagher, 2009; Greig, Taylor & MacKay, 2007; Rhodes, 2005). On these terms, research participants must be well informed and free from any controlling influences; researchers should do no harm and their overall influence should be beneficial; and research should be for the good of society as a whole, not just one privileged group – Aryan, in the case of the Third Reich.

Of the three key research principles, arguably the most contentious is a commitment to the good of society. Certainly it is the one principle that, in research ethics, failed to retain the original status given to it in the Nuremberg Code. Rhodes (2005), for example, noted how concern about serious inequality and injustice have been weakly interpreted in current research ethics as the necessity for obtaining informed consent, rather than ensuring that all research will be inclusive in its social benefit. Since Nuremberg, justice is addressed according to whether political emphasis is placed on the storyline of the "is" of particularised circumstances, brought alive through people's senses, or the "ought" of generalised aspirations, expressed through rationalisation and maximisation. Complex relationships of power direct the flow of these arguments, whose interweavings offer opportunities for interruptions, resistances and evasions.

These interweavings have produced several interpretations of (social) justice, and NZAC has over the years engaged with these ideas in various ways. Initially, following the example of biomedical ethics, many professional codes leaned towards this principled, universalistic position. The 1991 NZAC ethical code proposed a *principle* of *justice.* General Principle 4 stated: "counsellors shall be committed to the fair and equitable distribution of counselling services to all individuals and groups. Counsellors shall promote social justice through advocacy and empowerment" (NZAC, 1991, p. 1). The problem with this principled/universalist stance is the invitation to reduce all cultural and individual difference to rigid and fixed categories. In the revised NZAC Code (2002), the emphasis shifts to a core *value* of *social* justice, alongside an increased emphasis on Treaty responsibilities and "respect for individual and cultural differences and the diversity of human experience" (4.1). This goes some way towards discouraging counsellors from making static generalisations about clients and their various cultures, and encourages them to think about the various and multiple positions and group memberships that each individual may hold (see Margaret Agee et al., Part 1, Section 3).

These debates become important to ethical practice in counselling, in large part because of the emphasis in counselling on the uniqueness of, and thus difference between, persons: Rogers' (1962) argument for the prizing of persons is central to the history of the counselling profession, whatever theoretical paths people might have taken in the years since. An emphasis on prizing individuals and their uniqueness stands behind values such as autonomy (3.3). An associated emphasis on respecting difference, individual and cultural, is embodied in the principles of acting "with care and respect for individual and cultural differences and the diversity of human experience" (4.1). However, neither autonomy nor respecting difference and diversity are neutral concepts: both entangle counsellors in ambivalent relationships with power (Fairclough, 1992). The various positions that might be taken in order to maintain a commitment to both the "is" of the individual client and to the "ought" of social justice have been, and are still, dialogued vigorously among theorists.

Prizing individuals is not a single solution, and the resultant focus on personal power has often been blamed for the de-politicisation of therapy (Chantler, 2005). Counsellors still need to acknowledge group membership, which enables people to make claims on social justice. This perspective is often referred to as "identity politics" which, although a potent vehicle for change, has also been critiqued for making light of intra-group differences (for example, Bondi, 1993). More recently, and in order to avoid some of these critiques, the liberal humanistic concept of working with difference and diversity has become a dominant theme in the social services (for example, D'Cruz, 2007), and yet, that too has its critique. Chantler (2005) wrote:

> Whilst the promise of 'working with difference/diversity' was to counter the drawbacks of identity politics, and to move away from the notion of 'hierarchy' of oppressions, the reality has been quite different. Diversity has come to represent a diluted, more watered down approach, decontextualised and dislocated from the structures of power and privilege. (p. 241)

What has become increasingly apparent is that the various storylines and relationships of power intertwine in ways that call for different ways of thinking about individuals and their social context. Instead of focusing on one or the other, various new theoretical storylines suggest that it is more profitable to look at the ways in which personal and social storylines interweave – intersectionality – and position clients differently in relation to power at different times in their own lives, including at different moments. At which times does a client draw strength from her position as woman? When is it advantageous to identify as Pasifika? When does ability become a disadvantage? How does any one client navigate among the multiple positions available in the various contexts of everyday life? Of particular interest to counsellors are the times at which clients experience disadvantage through their exclusion from, or position within, any social grouping – minoritisation. Consequently, Chantler (2005) suggested that counsellors need to be aware of the dynamic processes of intersectionality and minoritisation when thinking about the power relationships between themselves, their clients and the rest of society.

THE STORYLINE OF PARTNERSHIP AND THE TREATY OF WAITANGI

These considerations are particularly poignant in revisiting Treaty responsibilities. As part of a commitment to social justice, NZAC has grappled with the implications of the Treaty of Waitangi for counsellors and counselling. The 2002 version of the *Code of Ethics* introduced partnership as a core value, partially to embrace the principles of protection, participation and partnership with Māori referred to in the introduction to the Code (Crocket, 2009; see Winslade, 2002). This is a brave move and situates counsellors in New Zealand differently from those in any other country. It moves beyond debates about sameness and difference and has real potential for a more respectful, sensitive, politically aware and relational form of ethics. The evolution of bicultural awareness in Aotearoa New Zealand has influenced thinking about social justice in this country and enabled us to make a unique contribution to international debates. Some implications of these commitments are discussed by Joy Te Wiata and Alastair Crocket earlier in Part 1 of this book.

Different counselling communities have taken different positions in relation to social justice and working with difference. For example, reflecting CACREP's (the Council for Accreditation of Counseling and Related Educational Programs)[1] professional standards for counsellor education in the USA, Corey, Corey and Callanan's (2007) general ethics text has an early chapter on "multicultural perspectives and diversity issues." In contrast, diversity and social justice are not highlighted anywhere in Barnes and Murdin's (2001) edited United Kingdom ethics text, which features psychodynamically-oriented or -derived perspectives. While both texts have the potential to contribute to the practice of ethics in an Aotearoa New Zealand setting, we cite this difference because we think it is important to notice which aspects of ethical practice particular texts, and particular professional communities, direct our attention to, and which aspects they do not consider.

Social justice is named as a core value in the NZAC *Code of Ethics*, and its expression is further elaborated upon in the principles and guidelines that follow, and in particular in Section 5.2, Respecting Diversity and Promoting Social Justice. Many authors in this book discuss aspects of ethics and social justice. For example, Colin Hughes, in considering

1 CACREP is the regulatory body that oversees counsellor education programmes in the USA.

the work of a school counsellor in the context of a wider pastoral care network (See Part 3, Section 3), draws attention to the complex matter of a counsellor's responsibility for the confidences of a young Māori woman. A school counsellor might need to weigh up the respecting of individual confidences with promoting the safety and well-being of whānau, and being honest and trustworthy in professional relationships.

The value of social justice is an expression of a wider ethos shared by members of the profession that goes beyond the particular work of individual counsellors. As members of professional communities we are each shaped and formed in the practice of ethics by all the communities of which we are part, and we each contribute to the shaping and forming of those communities. Thus, ethics is not just about the individual actions of individual practitioners, but about the particular ideas and practices that are made possible or not possible within particular professional cultures.

On the basis of their study of the experiences of workers in three Canadian social service sites, Rossiter, Prilleltensky, and Walsh-Bowers (2000) suggested that the separation of politics from ethics led to the marginalisation of ethics in all three sites. Rossiter et al. went on to argue for an understanding of ethics as part of the social organisation of agencies, rather than limiting our understanding of ethics to the actions of individual practitioners. Arguing for an "inherent connection between ethics and freedom" (p. 98), they suggested that conditions for dialogue, for democratic communication, are critical in centralising ethics in professional practice. These arguments contain echoes of those made locally by Webb (1998) who urged the profession to pay attention to the practices we select to replicate from the wider culture. If individual counsellors are to enact the principles of social justice, and to work in relation to the Code's guidelines on respecting diversity and promoting social justice, it would seem to us critical that counsellors continue to work to keep conversations about ethics and power woven through all daily professional practices: in meetings with clients, in our agencies, in supervision, and in wider professional forums.

1.5
MAKING DECISIONS FOR ETHICAL ACTION

Kathie Crocket

> In our view ... ethics is best protected when professionals perceive as their professional duty the responsibility to create relations of intersubjective respect. (Rossiter, Prilleltensky & Walsh-Bowers, 2000, p. 99)

This book's emphasis is the embeddedness of ethics in all the actions of our daily professional practices, coming from an orientation Bond (2010) referred to as "ethical mindfulness" (p. 242). Because of the professional relational responsibilities of our practice, it is incumbent on us to be able to account for these decisions and actions. This responsibility applies even when the processes and steps of our thinking, experiencing, and acting may not need to have the kinds of visibility they have when we are making overtly deliberate ethical decisions, such as whether or not to maintain a client's privacy, for example. This section sets out some commonly understood steps in making decisions for ethical action.

While it is common practice to talk about models of ethical decision-making, or as Bond (2010) describes it, ethical problem-solving, it is important to note that putting ethics into practice involves us in more than a technical process of decision-making, at a moment when some particularly sticky or tricky situation arises. In the various sections of Part 1 of this book we make some important points about the conditions for making decisions for ethical practice:

- Ethical action starts with skills and attitudes of ethical sensitivity in everyday practice;

- The ethical value of social justice interweaves ethics and politics;
- The New Zealand Association of Counsellors has chosen to name Treaty of Waitangi responsibilities within the *Code of Ethics* (2002);
- Ethical practice depends not only upon the actions of individual counsellors but also upon communities;
- Research suggests that practitioners value conditions for dialogue to support them in ethical practice (Rossiter et al., 2000).

In Part 3 of this book, Bill Grant argues for the importance of paying ongoing attention to affect in counselling. Ethical concerns can come out of and produce strong feelings such as commitment, fear, compassion, solidarity, anxiety, anger, blame, or shame. Our processes of engaging with both the ethics of daily practice and particular identified ethical concerns should include quality attention to the discomforts or unease we experience, including, as Hawkins (1997) reported, a sense of "not wanting to know" what the unease might be alerting us to.

With these points in mind, what follows are some particular practices that contribute to making purposeful decisions for ethical action. Although these practices are presented in a linear way, the processes will likely be recursive and organic:

> ... decisions are usually not made exclusively through a process of skilled deductive reasoning. Many other factors are also involved when we make important decisions about our own lives or the lives of others. ... Moral choice is an act of the whole person: it should involve all our mental faculties – reason, intuition, emotion, imagination – working in concert. (Hawkins, 1997, pp. 153–4)

1. Noticing an ethical question or concern

People report noticing ethical questions in different ways. Some would say that they have a practice of asking themselves about how power is being played out in relationship. Others might first notice a sense of embodied unease, which may not even have a name or location until they give it attention. However the concern comes to our notice, the next step is to turn towards it, to reach past any not-wanting-to-know (Hawkins, 1997) that might interrupt potential inquiry. A useful question might be: How is relationship being disturbed here?

2. Exploring the wider context of the question or concern
   - What is particular in this context that brings this question or concern to my attention?
3. Exploring the relationship between myself – my beliefs and values, my experiences, my theories of practice – and the question or concern
   - How might I map out the various dimensions on paper, through art or movement, on a computer, or in dialogue?
4. Naming and describing the concern on the basis of these explorations
   - How succinctly and clearly can I present the concern?
   - What remains unclear or confusing?
5. Documenting the process appropriately
   - What is wise for me to record in any professional notes in order to value the exploration?
6. Consulting the knowledge of my professional communities, including knowledge available in books, and the knowledge that is generated in dialogue with others. Possible reading includes:
   - the *Code of Ethics* of my own professional association;
   - other related codes of ethics (many available on-line);
   - my agency code of practice;
   - general ethics texts, and recent articles about the particular ethical matter;
   - Ludbrook's (2003) overview of counselling and the law in New Zealand; Part 4 of the current book for Simon Jefferson's contributions on the intersections of ethics and the law;
   - particular legislation such as the Privacy Act (1993);
   - my employment contract.

   People I might consult include my supervisor, a cultural consultant, colleagues, my manager, a member of the Ethics Committee, an ethicist from another discipline, in some instances another client or clients (while maintaining my ethical responsibilities in respect of privacy and confidentiality).

7. If the ethical concern is focused on my work with a particular client, perhaps I might consult directly with my client. Hill, Glaser and Harden (1998) and Walden (2006) suggested that a client be consulted at each step of the process, Walden arguing that such consultation is more likely to produce decisions that benefit of the client.

8. I might ask myself whether this concern appears to be one of those that is legalistic, that has me reaching first towards rules, or whether its central focus is relational, and has me reaching first towards thinking in terms of relational and moral responsibilities.

9. Going back to my own professional association's *Code of Ethics*, and reviewing the concern again in the light of values, principles and guidelines. Clarifying the concern, and possible and preferred responses, taking into account both my intentions and possible effects for others and for myself.

10. Inviting a senior professional to engage with me in caringly rigorous exploration of my proposed action in the light of my values, my intentions, and possible effects, and the values of relevant communities.

11. Taking responsive action in collaboration with others who support my purposes or share the responsibilities I carry.

12. Reviewing the effects of my actions and their implications and meanings, both in self-reflection and in consultation with others with whom I have already consulted, including, where appropriate, my client.

13. Reviewing the implications for my ongoing practice, and sharing that with others in my professional community.

There are many approaches to and models of ethical problem-solving and decision-making available in the ethics literature (Cottone & Claus, 2000). Cottone's (2001, 2004) particular contribution has been to re-focus ethical decision-making as a social and relational process rather than as an individual and intra-psychic process: "there is no individual decision-maker, because all decisions are made in the context of social interaction" (Cottone, 2004, p. 7).

For each of us, our selected approach to the practice of making particular ethical decisions is likely to be influenced by many factors, including our chosen practice approach, our ethno-cultural identification, or our experience with particular general decision-making practices, for example. And for all of us, making decisions about the ethics of practice will go on day by day, moment by moment, in the course of our everyday work, without the kinds of elaborated processes detailed here. But it is nonetheless important to have at hand an outline of a process, and a plan for careful and rigorous consultation, and consideration for those significant ethical concerns and questions that produce particular uncertainty, and that challenge us at the centre of the values we stand for in our practice.

1.6
USING A CODE OF ETHICS AS A WORKING DOCUMENT

Kathie Crocket

An aspirational code of ethics, such as NZAC's, articulates those shared values and ethical principles that a community of professional practice has agreed upon; offers guidelines for practice; and encourages ongoing ethical thinking and practice. The NZAC *Code of Ethics* is aspirational in its focus on values and principles and its restraint from stipulating rules (Winslade, 2002). It takes this form on the basis that we cannot know in advance how any particular situation will unfold:

> the challenge is how professional ethics might cover all members of a profession, be explicit and public, while at the same time guiding and supporting individual practitioners in making ethical sense of decisions between competing possible ethical actions. (Hugman, 2005, p. 148)

When we agree to abide by and aspire to such a code, the responsibility for interpretation and practice is taken by each of us in action in our professional work, in the context of local and professional community. This responsibility is one good reason for codes of ethics to be used as working documents which we consult regularly as we reflect on our practice: as we prepare to meet clients, as we encounter questions in agency practice or in third party work, as we prepare for supervision, as we write referral letters. A paper copy of our own professional association's code of ethics should be within reach in our practice rooms, and available to clients.

This suggestion, that codes of ethics are seen as working documents, does not come out of an interest in a rule-following approach to practice. Rather, it comes out of the idea that it is in the to and fro of relationship – in the to and fro of conversations with clients, with professional colleagues, supervisors and consultants, and in the to and fro of our own ongoing engagement with this working document – that we produce ethical practice. Ethics is action in the everyday relational work of practitioners: we are supported in that everyday work by familiarity with the statements of shared values and principles, and the guidelines for practice, that a code of ethics offers.

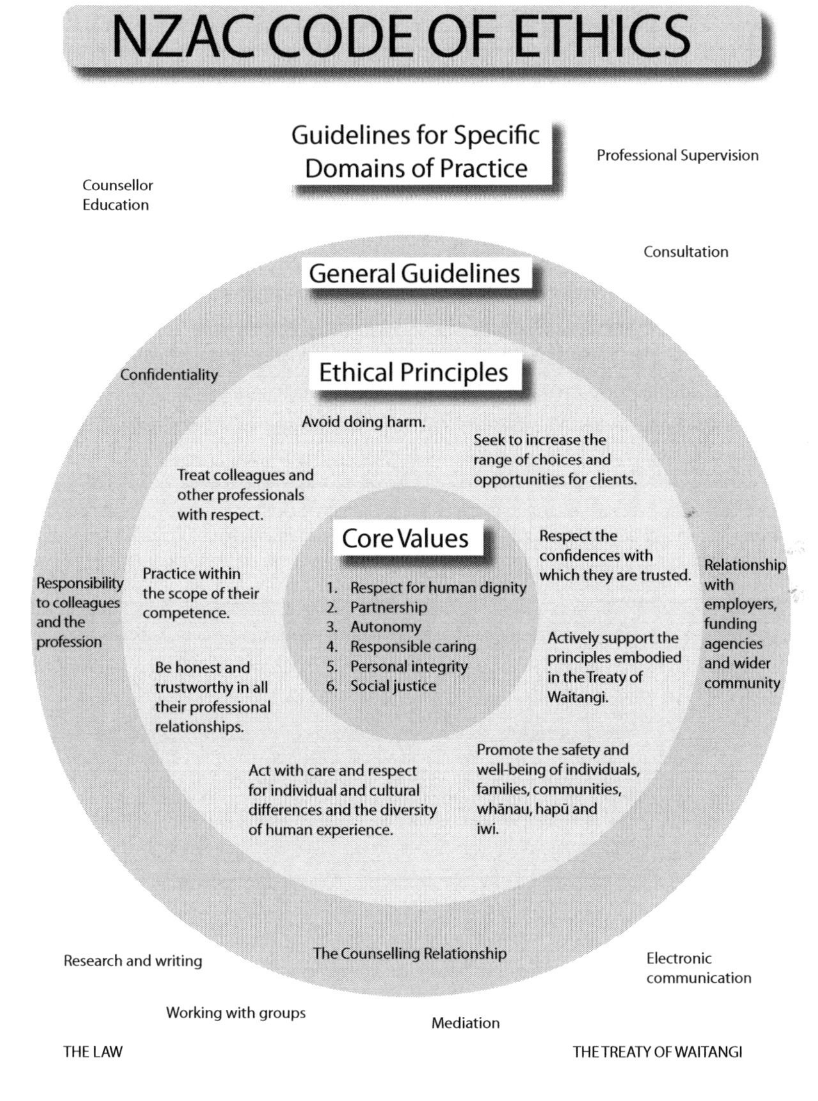

This diagram illustrates how at the heart of the NZAC *Code of Ethics* (NZAC, 2002) is a set of core values. Surrounding these values are a number of principles that also express these values. The values and principles are then expressed in a number of general guidelines that apply across various domains of counselling. Augmenting these general guidelines are guidelines for specific domains of practice. Thus, for a counsellor engaging in group work, for example, Core Values, Ethical Principles, General Guidelines, and the Guidelines specific to Group Work all apply (see Winslade, 2002). The NZAC *Code of Ethics* thus offers counsellors four embedded sites from which to consider the ethics of our practice: guidelines relating to specific practice, general guidelines, ethical principles, and core values of counselling. We should be familiar with this structure so that we consider the perspectives offered from each of these sites as we shape the ethics of our practice.

As the introduction to the NZAC *Code of Ethics* states, these considerations are all nested within the legislative context of the wider culture, and the Treaty of Waitangi:

> This Code needs to be read in conjunction with the Treaty of Waitangi and New Zealand law. Counsellors shall seek to be informed about the meaning and implications of the Treaty of Waitangi for their work. They shall understand the principles of protection, participation and partnership with Maori. Counsellors shall also take all reasonable steps to be informed about New Zealand law relevant to their work. (1)

PART 2

PRESENTING OURSELVES AS PROFESSIONALS

2.1 MARKETING, ADVERTISING AND ETHICS: COMMUNICATING WITH THE PUBLIC

Judi Miller

In the current competitive environment, we counsellors can find ourselves needing to consider the most effective ways of communicating with prospective clients. While this may be vital from a business perspective for practitioners who are self-employed, it may be just as necessary from an altruistic perspective for counsellors in other settings. Advertising may be the best way to provide information about counselling to groups within the community, to educate others about our role, and to offer information about access to counselling services. Here, I consider some ethical dilemmas inherent in advertising and marketing counselling services when the needs of both counsellors and their clients are taken into account.

WHAT GUIDANCE DO WE GET FROM CODES OF ETHICS?

Advertising is a well-known marketing technique, but neither NZAC nor the New Zealand Association of Psychotherapists (NZAP) makes direct statements about the ethics of advertising. Broad guidelines set by NZAC allow counsellors to use their own text to attract customers/clients but restrict the use of the Association's name, logo and letterhead (NZAC, 2002). Counsellors are given guidelines about advertising professional credentials correctly, including membership status, qualifications, training and competencies (7.3.g); setting and taking fees (5.6); contracting with clients about cancelled appointments and confidentiality (5.4.a); and are instructed not to solicit testimonials from current or former clients (5.12.b). They are also warned against exploiting their position within an organisation to recruit clients for their private practice (7.3.h), which would include avoiding unethical practices such as promoting courses that one is running for personal profit with one's own agency clients or students (see also 10.5.a). Similarly, NZAP members are instructed to restrain their commercial self-interest by adhering to professional standards in conducting their practices, advertising services, and setting fees that are reasonable (NZAP, 2008). Furthermore, the New Zealand Psychological Society's (NZPSS) Code instructs members not to exploit any work relationship to further their own personal or business interests (NZPSS, 2002).

These general guidelines are similar to those of international counselling associations. The ACA *Code of Ethics,* however, specifically mentions advertising and gives specific advice, such as regular checking that electronic links are working and professionally appropriate (ACA, 2005, A.12.h.1).

WHAT ARE SOME ETHICAL DILEMMAS ASSOCIATED WITH COUNSELLOR ADVERTISING?

1. The ethos of counselling – caring, helping empathising, empowering and facilitating growth – seems at odds with the commercial world of profit, consumption and promotion. Leicht and Fennell (2001) noted the difference between collective goals for accountability and efficiency, and individual expectations. Individual clients seek professional services that they know and trust, with a person they can meet face-to-face regularly. As counsellors, therefore, we must balance our views on marketing our services with our views of potential clients' needs to see and talk with the person who will be providing their service.
2. Many counsellors serve at least two client groups: the clients who require counselling and third-party funding agencies. This exposes the ethical and representational dilemmas inherent in needing to present oneself in two or more different ways. Davis and Freeman (1996) noted that third-party funding agencies want professionalism, consultation and prompt return of reports, but individuals and families want understanding, unconditional regard, respect, empathy and consideration. Obviously, advertising that emphasises the needs of one party (for efficient production of reports) could be unattractive to the other (Kotler & Bloom, 1984).

3. Counsellors offer a service that cannot be seen in advance of purchase, making it more difficult for clients to evaluate than a material product. Furthermore, the harder a product is to evaluate in advance of purchase or use, the greater the perceived risk for the customer. The marketing techniques used by counsellors should, therefore, aim to offer clear information relevant to clients' potential concerns about the counselling they might receive (Lovelock, Patterson & Walker, 1998).

4. Related to this is the issue of the vulnerability of some client groups. It behoves us to take care not to exaggerate or misrepresent our professional skill, competence and qualifications, or the potential outcomes of our service, especially when we consider client factors such as poverty, knowledge gaps, and other forms of vulnerability.

5. Exaggeration carries the potential for doing harm. Let us consider this example from an online advertisement and decide if the client's perceived risk is addressed: "Experience happiness, joy, freedom! Offering professional counselling for emotional well-being, substance abuse and recovery, anxiety or depression, and relationship issues. Discover your own inner strength and solutions." (http://www.kasamba.com/advice/browse). As well as being unethical, such claims may be in breach of the Advertising Standards Authority and its *Code of Practice*.

6. Using the internet to communicate with potential clients expands risks associated with client confidentiality, verification of counsellor credentials, and counsellor accessibility during technological failure. The ACA *Code of Ethics* has several pertinent suggestions to protect consumer rights and facilitate addressing relevant ethical concerns. Examples include the need to provide a site that is accessible to persons with disabilities (A.12.h.6), that contains translation capabilities for clients who have a different primary language (A.12.h.7), and that assists clients to determine the validity and reliability of WWW material (A.12.h.8).

WHAT INFORMATION SHOULD COUNSELLORS PROVIDE?

The dilemmas listed above highlight the need for counsellors to consider, carefully, their intended purpose when advertising, in light of their own needs and the needs and rights of their clients. Promoting informed choices for clients, Manthei and Miller (2000) listed the following as useful information:

- title, qualifications and training;
- experience of working with specific problems;
- professional association and *Code of Ethics*;
- supervision;
- professional development;
- fees;
- estimate of time in counselling;
- insurance payments;
- length of session;
- cancellation policies;
- model of counselling used;
- policy on confidentiality, record keeping and complaints procedures.

In addition, it may be helpful to include relevant information about counsellors' cultural identities and affiliations, such as ethnicity, languages spoken, sexual identity, and so on. This is consistent with clause 5.2.g in the NZAC *Code of Ethics* regarding the equitable provision of counselling services to all individuals and social groups.

When I analysed a small sample of counsellor advertising brochures (Miller, 2003), I found that many counsellors included the information recommended by Manthei and Miller (2000), as well as photographs and some personal information. Care is needed when including personal information. While it may be used to emphasise a counsellor's belief that their family composition, church affiliation or parenthood makes them accessible and trustworthy, it may also appear to disrespect the diversity of clients (5.2). Information about the counsellor's cultural affiliations may, however, help potential clients make informed decisions about their counselling. The common omissions in counsellor advertising brochures were information about the process of counselling, what clients could expect from it, and the meaning of terms such as "experience," "confidentiality" and/or "supervision". Inclusion of these aspects, would not only help clients evaluate a product before purchase (Lovelock et al., 1998) but also complies with ethical guidelines to communicate to clients the extent and limits of confidentiality (6.1.c) and the purpose, risks, limits and costs of counselling (5.5.b).

In terms of ethical guidelines, counsellors in New Zealand are restricted very little in their advertising. If we are thinking about clients' perspectives, and respecting their rights, however, I would suggest that we consider carefully how we use advertising in marketing our services. When we promote ourselves as caring and supportive listeners who are accountable and experienced, we are asking clients to enter our services by trusting us as professionals (Miller, 2003). When we promise clients self-actualisation, fulfilment and personal growth, we are asking them to favourably dispose themselves to our product. While both types of advertising are ethical, it is advisable to advertise within the ethical principle of counselling to "be honest and trustworthy in all professional relationships" (4.7). Marketing that focuses on characteristics that can be substantiated satisfies this ethical principle.

2.2 PROFESSIONAL DISCLOSURE STATEMENTS

Judi Miller

A professional disclosure statement informs a prospective client about the qualifications of a counsellor and the nature of the counselling process so that a client is able to make an informed decision regarding the use of a counsellor's services (Gill, 1982). A disclosure statement is more than a fact sheet and has the following benefits:

- Giving information about counselling to clients prior to their first session can have a beneficial impact on the counselling process, by facilitating the engagement process (Gill, 1982);
- It can contribute to the genuineness and congruence necessary for effective helping relationships because it models transparency (Gill, 1982);
- It has the potential to enhance the image of the counselling profession (see Miller, 2003);
- It communicates respect for clients and promotes a context in which the session will be seen as valuable (Coles, 1995);
- It may increase client attendance rates (Coles, 1995).

WRITING A PROFESSIONAL DISCLOSURE STATEMENT

Gill (1982) posed very useful questions to help guide the writing of these statements. These guidelines fall into three categories:

1. Information about the counsellor, including: credentials in relation to the service provided; professional development and supervision arrangements; professional membership; which clients might benefit; and counsellor beliefs about what helps people lead more satisfying lives;
2. Information about the process: what a client might expect; the approach, methods, strategies and techniques that might be used, and why; the confidential nature of counselling, and client rights, including a complaints process; and how a client might prepare for counselling;
3. Administrative matters: policy about fees, hours, cancellations.

SOME ETHICAL CONSIDERATIONS RELEVANT TO THE USE OF PROFESSIONAL DISCLOSURE STATEMENTS

1. The ethical guidelines that apply to counsellor advertisements also apply to professional disclosure statements (see Part 2, Section 1).
2. For reasons of confidentiality or client safety it is important to check before posting your professional disclosure statement to a prospective client.
3. If your statement is a form of contract, it will be important to take steps to clarify the detail of what you are asking a client to agree to.
4. A statement should be clear and accessible in language and content.

An exemplar of a professional disclosure statement

Counselling Centre logo/address

Dear ...

This letter is to introduce myself to you, welcome you to the counselling centre and give you some information about what to expect when you come for your appointment.

I am a counsellor with a background in xx. I am a member of the New Zealand Association of Counsellors, a professional organisation with a code of ethics, and a complaints process.

At this centre we provide a professional and confidential service. We take your safety seriously. At our first meeting, which will last for about an hour, I will be interested in getting to know you a little and we can talk about the things that concern you. I will be happy to tell you more about my experience, qualifications and supervision arrangements. We will talk together about how many sessions we will meet for and how often we will review the progress of counselling and your satisfaction.

My standard fee is xx per hour, to be paid at the beginning of each session. If you are unable to attend, or wish to change an appointment time, please let me know by giving me at least 24 hours notice to allow me to offer your time to someone else. If you don't come to a session but have not let me know in advance that you will not be coming, I will charge you half of the normal fee for that missed session.

As a way of preparing for our first session, I would like you to think about what you are hoping to get out of counselling. Some of the things I will be curious about are:

[*List here questions that reflect your approach to counselling. For example: What are your main concerns? How long have these been a worry? What effects do they have on you and your relationship? Or: What are your concerns? How have you tried to solve them? If there have been any improvements since you contacted me, what have you noticed that you have been doing differently?*]

My hope is that I can help you find some ideas or directions that fit with you, and encourage you to use your own knowledge and abilities to gain the change you want.

I'm looking forward to meeting you at ... ... on ... . here at the centre. There is a car park and bike rack behind the building and a bus stop right outside. Please come in the front door, where our receptionist will greet you.

2.3
THE SETTING FOR COUNSELLING: PRIVATE PRACTICE

Fran Parkin and Kathie Crocket

Private, or independent, practice involves counselling in the context of one's own business, including taking responsibility for ethical, organisational, and business aspects of a counselling practice. This includes those aspects nominated by Syme (1994): "accepting referrals, counselling clients in one's own time, using one's own premises and charging a fee" (p. 6). Private practice takes a variety of forms: sole practice or group practice; independent or in association with another service; and full-time, part-time, or a very limited occasional practice alongside other employment. In each of these forms, careful consideration should be given to the particular ethical dimensions of private practice.

An increasing proportion – currently more than 30 percent – of NZAC members identify themselves as being in private practice (NZAC, 2010), a trend also noted in Cornforth and Sewell's (2004) study of the graduates of polytechnic counsellor education programmes. This trend was investigated by Manthei, Rich, Agee, Monk, Miller, Bunce, Webb, and Hermansson (1994), and Paton (1995, 1999, 2005), who suggested that private practitioners reported mostly positive effects in terms of lifestyle, reduced stress, and increased autonomy. These authors also highlighted tensions to be addressed in terms of overall ethical responsibilities to clients and the profession. This section draws on this New Zealand research, considering, first, ethical responsibilities for ensuring the appropriateness of entering private practice; and second, ethical aspects of presenting oneself as a professional in private practice, including the physical setting, and policies and practices. It concludes with scenarios for reflection.

EVALUATING THE APPROPRIATENESS OF PRIVATE PRACTICE

There are some significant aspects of presenting oneself as a professional that should be considered before setting up in any form of private practice. Noting that in private practice "there is no employer to hire counsellors of an appropriate standard and to fire those who behave unprofessionally," Syme (1994, p. 12) suggested that a counsellor needs at least ten years' experience before taking on the particular responsibilities of private practice. This recommendation serves as a caution to practitioners about the seriousness of the responsibilities of private practice. Length of experience is but one dimension to consider in assessing whether private practice is an appropriate setting. The following questions may provide a useful starting point to evaluate, in discussion with supervisors and other professional colleagues, the appropriateness, or not, of a move into private practice.

- What experiences do I bring to support me as a private practitioner?
- What resources do I have to call on if I am to present myself as a professional in a private practice?
- What about vulnerabilities for myself and those I might work with?
- Is this the right time in my professional career, and in my personal life, for me to be considering a private practice option?
- Who would support me in this move? Why would they support me?
- Who would caution me against this move? Why would they caution me?
- What are the particular features of the kind of private practice I am proposing, and what are the implications of these features for ethical practice?
- Would private practice be a context where, at this time in my career, I can confidently practice in terms of the stated ethical values and principles of the NZAC *Code of Ethics* (2002), including practising within the scope of my competence (4.8)?

THE LOCATION OF PRIVATE PRACTICE

Some private practitioners work in a group practice, agency, or health setting, with either a partnership or company structure; some work on their own in independent premises where they may or may not undertake contracted work for agencies and third-party funders; and some counsellors work from a home-based practice. Each of these contexts raises particular ethical questions.

The NZAC *Code of Ethics* states that counsellors "assume full responsibility for setting and monitoring boundaries between a counselling relationship with a client and any other kind of relationship and for making such boundaries as clear as possible to the client" (5.11.a). Counsellors working in private practice from home face particular ethical challenges to do with the separation of home and work. There is potential for benefit to the counselling relationship, and also for harm. In a home office context it is more difficult to maintain privacy, and clients will inevitably form some responses to personal circumstances that may influence the counselling relationship. Clients are much more likely to make assumptions about marital status, family situation, economic status, and even political interests by coming into a home space. Such assumptions need to be anticipated to minimise potentially harmful effects. Relevant considerations for protecting the privacy of both clients and counsellors include:

- clear separation of home and personal space;
- separation of landlines, mobile phones, answer phones and email addresses for private/household use and professional use;
- signage;
- appropriate waiting areas;
- sound protection between counselling and waiting rooms, and the rest of the house;
- access to toilets.

These matters need forethought in a group practice, too. The approach to the building; how the waiting room is decorated; posters on a notice board; magazines or books, all potentially influence the counselling relationship even before a client enters the counselling room. Then there is the furnishing of the room, aesthetically and in terms of physical comfort. If we are to work in terms of the NZAC *Code of Ethics'* call to respect diversity, we may want to think about the effects of our private practice environments for people of different cultures, genders or sexual orientations, as well as in terms of physical access. Attention to physical safety, such as evacuation procedures, is also relevant.

ESTABLISHING POLICIES AND PROCEDURES

Agencies offer the counsellors they employ clear policies and procedures designed to assist professional conduct and ethical practice. Counsellors working in private practice, as individuals or in group practice, should also develop clear policies and procedures that incorporate ethical values and principles, as well as mechanisms to ensure that these policies and procedures are regularly evaluated and revised. We suggest that policies should cover the following basic areas, which include both practical and ethical considerations.

Scope of practice What is the focus of your practice, given the competencies you have? How do you access clients? The NZAC *Code of Ethics* stipulates that counsellors "determine, in consultation with their client, whether they are appropriate to provide counselling," including "by reason of skills, gender, or culture" (5.3). What assessment and contracting processes do you use? What are your referral procedures, both in terms of the agencies that refer to you, and those to which you refer?

Contracting and assessment These processes are particularly important in private practice. Establishing the purpose for the initial visit on the phone when making an appointment; engaging in a thorough mutual initial assessment of the problem a client brings; and having a clear understanding of counselling expectations, including those of a referral agency, are important steps. These steps assess the appropriateness of any particular counselling relationship and establish agreed understandings of the purpose of counselling.

Workload and availability The management of workload is a particular challenge of private practice, particularly when a counsellor's income is dependent upon the numbers of clients seen in a week. Planning is therefore very important.

What are your hours of practice? How many hours do you work with clients each week? When do you attend to other aspects of your business? How do clients make contact with you outside appointment times? When do you respond to phone messages? How far in advance do you plan the workload and financial management involved in taking holidays?

Storage of notes Paper records should be in lockable storage, and computers should be password protected (see Part 3, Sections 1, 2 and 14) Arrangements should be made, too, for who would have access to take care of your client records in the event of your being unable to do so yourself.

Safety What procedures do you have in place in the event of having to respond to violence or other intention to harm? (See Part 3, Section 17 for a discussion of counsellor responsibilities in such situations.)

Fees How do you manage your fee structure, missed appointments, cancellations, debts, and pro-bono work? What matters do you take into account when you reduce fees, or defer payments? It is considered wise practice to consult with a supervisor, and to have a clear rationale, in situations where a counsellor goes outside their usual practice in respect of fees.

Supervision, professional competence, fitness to practice, and professional-self-care The NZAC *Code of Ethics* refers to a number of ways in which to sustain and monitor professional practice. What arrangements do you have for regular supervision? Who supports you in making a professional development plan? How do you plan time and money for peer support, professional networking, and other professional contact?

There are particular responsibilities to colleagues and the profession that should be planned for. What arrangements do you have for monitoring your fitness to practice, or resolving any difficulties that might arise?

Medical backup and other referrals Clear referral arrangements support practice within the scope of your competence. What referral arrangements do you have for matters beyond your scope of practice or competence, including medical, mental health, community, and legal referrals?

Disclosure statements and advertising Are the claims you make an honest representation of your competence? (See Judi Miller, Part 2, Section 1.)

Informing clients of the availability of government funding Do you know about alternative funding and do you refer clients to appropriate alternative free or low-cost options, as advised in the NZAC *Code of Ethics* (2002, 5.2)?

Support for planned and unplanned absence from your practice Relational responsibilities for clients extend to planning for your absence. What arrangements do you make for planned absences such as holidays or professional development? What ongoing arrangements do you have in place for sudden, unexpected absence, such as illness, accident or death? Planning should include having the commitment from someone trustworthy, preferably another professional, to act as a "therapeutic executor" (Traynor & Clarkson, 1992, p. 23), to take responsibility in a situation of sudden, unexpected absence.

SOME PRACTICE SCENARIOS FOR REFLECTION

Home and work distinctions

You operate a private practice from your home office. You have ensured a separation of home and work by providing a separate entrance and waiting room, and separate home and work telephone lines. Your teenage son is washing his car out on the street. A client inquires about your son and what he does.

A counsellor is responsible for privacy considerations for both clients and their own family members. Such considerations should also be balanced with care and respect for individual differences. How a counsellor responds should take account of the potential for harm, and to whom, as well as the potential for building respect.

Safety for a counsellor

You are a female counsellor, alone in your private practice. A new male client reveals he has a problem with stalking. He says he wants help to resist his urges to masturbate while watching his female neighbour dressing and undressing.

Working on one's own, or in an isolated setting, can put private practitioners at some personal risk, including risk of false complaint. Protective measures that can be taken include a panic alarm, having someone else in the building, telephone assessment, and limiting one's client base. For example, some counsellors do not take Family Court referrals.

Safety for a client

A client struggling with depression reveals that she is feeling suicidal and has the means to carry out this threat. She does not want you to contact her family or the Mental Health Community Crisis Team.

Having a safety strategy in place is a critical aspect of suicide prevention and intervention. This may include medical or psychiatric back-up, working in co-operation with existing services a client may be using, and agreed back-up plans with colleagues and supervisors. It also certainly includes informed consent processes that make clear that exceptions to confidentiality include situations where there is imminent risk of serious harm (5.1.d, 6.2.c) (see also Margaret Agee, Part 3, Section 17).

Scope of practice

Your workload is currently light and you hold concern for the viability of your practice. A friend of a current client phones, saying she hears from her friend how helpful you have been. She asks if you can help her with an eating disorder. This is not a problem you have dealt with before.

Economic uncertainties can leave counsellors in private practice vulnerable to taking on referrals outside their competence. Any referrals need to be considered in the light of professional ethical responsibilities, particularly to avoid doing harm, and the availability of other funded or partially funded counselling services.

Setting fees

A client has a background in painting but doesn't have current employment as he cannot work full time. Your house needs painting and you haven't had time to find a painter. You wonder about exchanging counselling for painting.

The NZAC *Code of Ethics* states clearly that clients should not be exploited for financial gain (5.12.a); and cautions counsellors about accepting goods and services in lieu of payment (5.6.c). Fees and methods of payment should be set at the commencement of counselling, according to one's policies. Any change from one's normal practice should be a matter for consultation in supervision, and should have a clear professional rationale.

Undertaking appropriate professional development

Aspects of some current client practice are particularly stretching and you are noticing the professional isolation. Out of the blue, a colleague phones and invites you to join a peer consultation group for networking and support. The group seems to offer opportunities to maintain competent practice and fitness to practice (5.9, 5.10), through the relationships of professional and personal care it would foster. But these are tough economic times and there would be a cost of travel and lost working time to attend these fortnightly group meetings.

New Zealand private practice research (Manthei et al., 1994; Paton, 1995) emphasises the importance of supervision for reviewing both the practicalities and the psycho-social effects of a counsellor's workload, as well as the value of professional networks and peer support.

IN CONCLUSION

This section has largely taken an approach to the everyday practice of ethics that seeks to anticipate and prevent potential harm. In this way it is perhaps liability-focused. However, many practitioners engage in private practice in order to take responsibility for the immediate professional culture in which they work. In this way, private practice also offers counsellors rich opportunity to engage critically and reflexively in the ethical complexities of our moral responsibilities towards those we meet as clients.

2.4
WORKING BEYOND THE AGENCY WALLS

Jenny Snowdon

There is a wide diversity of opportunities for working beyond the agency walls. My own experience covers work in school interview rooms, meeting young people for hot chocolate in cafés, talking in the agency car park, visiting hospital rooms and going to meet families in their homes. In the interests of succinctness, I limit the scope of this chapter to meeting with people in their homes. Many of the ethical considerations I take up in this chapter will have application in other settings.

I meet with the Jackson/Morgan family in their home, after school. Prior to this meeting the family and I have discussed the options of meeting at the agency rooms or meeting in their home. On this occasion, Mary has asked that I come to their home because she believes her children will find it easier to talk to me "on their own turf." I have asked whether it will be easy or not so easy to set aside an hour or so from homework, TV, visitors and phone calls. Mary thinks everyone is pretty keen to talk to me and we have agreed together we will take responsibility for keeping our meeting focused on the concerns the family want to talk about. When I arrive, both Mary and Phil are home from work and they call their children from various parts of the house to the lounge.

When counsellors work beyond the agency walls, we align with the core value of partnership and with the ethical principle of the NZAC *Code of Ethics* that says we "seek to increase the range of choices and opportunities for clients" (NZAC, 2002, 4.6). Furthermore, counselling beyond the agency walls demands that counsellors respect the dignity and cultural diversity of those who consult us, in particular ways, when we enter their homes (4.1). In thinking about our work beyond the agency walls, I also bring forward an ethical commitment to social justice (3.6).

As a counsellor whose work sometimes takes me – in a spirit of partnership, collaboration and alliance – beyond the agency walls, I think about issues of social interaction that include:

RECOGNISING LIMITED RESOURCE

- What is the agency's commitment to social justice, and what is mine, in relation to limited resource?
- Does the family have access to a car and money for petrol?
- Are there matters of health, such as depression or panic attacks or cancer treatment, that make it difficult for a person to meet with me outside home at this time? Does the person have eyesight, hearing or mobility challenges that make it difficult to attend counselling sessions away from home?

We cannot sidestep considerations of inequity and injustice when we are asked to engage with people in therapeutic conversations (Waldegrave, 1990). When therapy takes a broad, ecological approach it can link therapeutic problems to cultural and socioeconomic contexts, a move towards "shared social concern" (Waldegrave, 1990, p. 24). Simply put, it may be that my visit to the family home makes it easier for them to meet a counsellor and this is reason enough to explore this option.

Mary and Phil sit quietly when the meeting starts. Despite the setting, their home, they place me in the speaker's chair. I take up the invitation and begin by asking questions of the members of the family by way of introduction/whakawhanaungatanga. I tell the family that my hope is that they will have questions for me in return. Jane (10) wants to know how old I am. This is followed by Carl's (7) interest in whether I have any children of my own. (If no questions had been asked, I would have spoken about my life in ways that allowed the family to suss me out and offered openings for curiosity on the part of family members.) Mary asks me if I would like a cup of tea since she is about to have one.

WELCOMING THE HOSPITALITY OF OTHERS

- When I remove my shoes and step into the place and cultural practices of people in their homes, how will I appreciate what is centrally important to the family as we meet? What opens up for them when they host the meeting rather than being the guests of the agency or private practice? As I enter a person's home and act with care and respect for difference and diversity, I appreciate anew the practice that becomes possible when I think of myself, in Aileen Cheshire's words, as a "guest" in that person's life (cited in Crocket, 2008).
- If, from time to time, my experience is of being on unfamiliar ground in places beyond the agency walls, can this inform my sensitivity to what it is like for people to enter my counselling room, and stand on unfamiliar ground? I propose that standing on unfamiliar ground offers me, as counsellor, opportunities for learning and experiencing differently the subtle shifts of power in the therapeutic relationship.
- An ethical question that sits with me when I meet with people at home (or school) is: now that I have been given a welcome here, how will I make it clear that home (or school) is not a place I will visit unannounced? I inform people that I will arrange my visits ahead of time.

Mary's daughter, Suze, wants to speak to me, so we negotiate a way for the rest of the family to listen without speaking for a time. I also wonder out loud if Suze wants a family audience or if she prefers to speak privately to me. In this case, Suze and I work out that I will ask seven questions to start with, and Suze nominates one of her siblings to keep an accurate count! In the course of talking with Suze, some troubling aspects of school life emerge and Suze, crying, goes to sit with her mother for a hug. In the past, Mary and Suze have had close alliances but these have been disintegrating. In this moment, a movement back towards "being on the same side" becomes possible again.

TAKING UP AND OFFERING SPEAKING POSITIONS IN RESPECTFUL PARTNERSHIP

- In what ways will it be possible for me to maintain my professional stance in a family home setting? I understand the interwoven nature of power relations in counselling work, so meeting beyond the agency walls does not mean I abdicate responsibility for guiding the conversation.
- Home settings may or may not be more inviting of conversation for children. Is there willingness, and room, for children to speak with a counsellor privately at home if children or their parent(s) want this to happen?
- Meeting families in their homes provides opportunities to engage with material aspects of their lives. For example, ready access to awards, created objects and artefacts of family life can be an advantage in forming the counselling partnership. When a family member speaks at home of her/his achievements with the counsellor, ready access to the actual item may make it possible to witness the story of achievement eloquently and closely.

My orientation in therapy includes an understanding that what I do will engage me with the family in political activity that has the potential to challenge expert knowledge and bring forward the person's knowledge (Epston, White & "Ben", 1995; White & Epston, 1990). There is something about the home environment that can make the playing field more even for acknowledging "local" knowledge. Reciprocity is important here. Counsellors are both giving and receiving in the counselling relationships we form, and this may be more readily visible when we meet at people's home. People may 'see' themselves as more authoritative about problems they want to deal with, and may find networks of support more accessible, when they speak in the very setting where new ways of living will be carried out. Hare-Mustin (1994) challenged counsellors to be mindful of the structural inequalities of therapeutic relationships. These challenges suggest that even if we meet beyond the agency walls, the discourses of the mirrored (counselling) room are reflected in the lounge-rooms of people's homes.

COUNSELLING BEYOND THE AGENCY WALLS REQUIRES AN EXTENSION OF COUNSELLOR COMPETENCY AND SKILLS

These competencies include the following:

- Phone contact and initial negotiation help prepare the family and begins an informed consent process. Negotiation will include: a suitable time and setting, who will attend the meeting, minimising and managing potential distractions ahead of time.
- Materials we will need to work together need to be prepared ahead.
- It is important to set the scene for how we will work, in general and in specific terms. For instance, we might put words to how this visit will be different from a visit by friends or neighbours. I ask questions about what the family hopes for from the counselling meeting, explain how I plan to involve the different family members in our conversation, and ask how this suits the family.
- Deferring to family practices whilst taking up professional responsibility, I ask, for example, whether anyone has plans following our meeting so that I can be courteous towards other commitments the family has.

Sometimes, home environments are not conducive to the kinds of ethical practice that I have described above. There are moments of interruption and distraction that lead people to prefer the set-aside place that a counsellor's room affords. People may prefer the otherness of the counselling agency setting in order to give space to alternative storylines of their lives. People may want the privacy of being in conversation with a counsellor away from usual living situations. A person may want to be offered hospitality by another. A person may want the setting for counselling to provide a clear boundary around the professional relationship in order to avoid the possibility of multiple relationships.

SAFETY FOR THE COUNSELLOR IS A PHYSICAL AND ETHICAL CONSIDERATION IN WORK BEYOND THE AGENCY WALLS

Working beyond the agency walls requires skills for managing potentially volatile situations: judging the risk to others and oneself; using words and tone of voice to calm a volatile situation; accessing immediate health/social work/legal support and police protection, if necessary. Practical guidelines and agency policy can support safety for counsellors:

- For example, a counsellor will park the car on the street; might use an unmarked car; and has available mobile phone contact with the agency;
- A counsellor, having assessed the current risk, may ask to postpone a meeting or renegotiate to meet at the agency rooms;
- A counsellor will inform colleagues and supervisors of a situation that is a safety concern.

Although this outline does not cover all contingencies, it points to ways of thinking about risk that take account of the welfare of self and others, and these count as ethical practices.

Working beyond the agency walls has important ethical implications for counselling practice and should always be undertaken in the interests of the person consulting us. When inequities and injustice are at play in the lives of people who consult us for therapy, going out to meet people in their homes provides recognition of the wider social concerns that impact lives, and invites us to participate differently to address unequal and unjust situations. We can no longer be oblivious to the obvious, when we see it for ourselves. Counsellors who meet people at home accept the hospitality of others, on their terms *and* on mutually negotiated terms. This move is one that can promote possibilities for consulting those who consult us, and allow reciprocity that might be more elusive in the agency setting. Not always. At every moment we engage in thinking ethically about what effects our actions will have.

2.5
SOLICITING CLIENTS

John Winslade

What kinds of marketing methods can counsellors use to solicit clients in private practice contexts? In this setting counsellors are clearly operating a business and sound business practices apply. But the business of counselling is also bound by the ethics that govern the delivery of a professional service, which makes higher demands in terms of standards than the trading of goods might require. Professions have a long history of altruism which sanctions baselines for behaviour more stringent than those of fair exchange in the marketplace. For example, the principle of *caveat emptor* (let the buyer beware) would not suffice as an ethical baseline for professional practice.

The NZAC *Code of Ethics* (2002) recognises these professional stringencies in its outline of a set of principles to govern the practice of counselling in New Zealand. Among other principles, counsellors are enjoined "to be honest and trustworthy in all their professional relationships" (4.7), to "practice within the scope of their competence" (4.8) and to "treat colleagues and other professionals with respect" (4.9). These principles would not be expressed, for example, through false advertising, through exaggerated claims of competence given to clients, or through negative comparative advertising which referred to other counselling services.

Within the specific guidelines that the NZAC *Code of Ethics* elaborates there are further implications that build upon these general principles. One of the headings is "responsibility to the profession" (7.3). This ethic of responsibility is specific to professions in a way that is different from the selling of goods (although there are examples of other forms of responsibility in those domains. Think for example of the responsibility of retailers to sell toys that are safe). But the public expects professionals to maintain a higher standard of trustworthiness than other businesses, and to do things for the public good rather than just for their own or their clients' benefit. Hence counsellors are expected to "represent honestly and accurately their membership status [within NZAC], their qualifications, training and competencies" (7.3.d). We are used to, and have become tolerant of, advertising methods that contain a degree of exaggeration by the use of vague-sounding words that can be taken to mean a range of things, but that suggest promises beyond those which the product can provide. In the interests of the profession, counsellors should err on the side of prudence and caution in what they claim.

Specifically, counselling should remain a service rather than a product in the ways we talk about it. Counsellors can make no guarantees about the outcomes of counselling. The principle of informed consent also enters this domain. Any hint of deception or exaggeration in processes of advertising or solicitation could be argued to infringe the right of the client to informed consent and to undermine the ethic of openness for the whole profession. For example, it would not be acceptable for a counsellor to introduce hidden costs that were submerged in the fine print of the original contract. Even if strictly legal, such practices could be interpreted as deceptive and in breach of the ethic of negotiating "clear and reasonable" contracts (5.4.a).

Another issue arises when counsellors are employed in an organisation, and, at the same time, maintain a private practice. Imagine, for example, a school counsellor who sees a child at school along with their parent. Is it acceptable for a counsellor to say to the two clients, "I don't have time to help you deal with this at school, but I could arrange to meet you in my private practice capacity"? The NZAC *Code of Ethics* prohibits counsellors from using their position in an organisation "to recruit clients for their own private practice" (7.3.e). Here, a conflict of interest is involved. The counsellor has a pecuniary interest in that private practice which clashes with the counsellor's responsibility as an employee to the organisation through which the clients have met the counsellor. The problem is that there is the potential for the suspicion that the counsellor is making this referral to him- or herself on the basis of self-interest rather than on a more altruistic basis.

At the heart of good counselling is the establishment of a profound experience of trust. NZAC certainly advocates for such a level of trust in its definition of what counselling is about. Professional standards need to be observed when soliciting clients. Counsellors are advised to be prudent, circumspect and cautious in the ways they go about recruiting clients.

2.6
TESTIMONIALS FROM CLIENTS

Margaret Agee

Using client testimonials, or sharing with others a spontaneous appreciative personal communication from a client, is likely to be ethically problematic. The NZAC *Code of Ethics* (2002, 5.4, 5.12b) explicitly prohibits counsellors from seeking testimonials from clients. While some clients or former clients would be sufficiently confident to exercise their autonomy in responding to such a request, and some would even be pleased to be asked, others may find it difficult, if not impossible, to refuse. Such a request runs the risk of exploiting a client's gratitude, and consciously or unwittingly pressuring a client to comply (5.12.a). Because of the inherent imbalance of power in the professional relationship between counsellor and client, and because of the possibility of a client holding a sense of obligation to the counsellor, a client or former client is making such a decision in a constrained relational environment. The fact that the counsellor is making a personal/professional request of the client in this professional context may also contribute to the potential for coercion, however carefully the counsellor may reassure the client that there is no pressure intended.

There is also the situation where a counsellor receives a spontaneous appreciative personal communication from a client. Such a message can be a source of deeply moving affirmation of a counsellors' sense of professional self-worth, bearing testimony to their effectiveness in enabling clients to make meaningful changes in their lives. The critical ethical points to consider here are privacy, informed consent, and relationships of power.

In commenting on such situations, Winslade (1998) pointed out that even the knowledge that a particular individual has seen a counsellor is considered private and personal information under the Health Information Privacy Code (1994), and should therefore not be disclosed without the consent of the client. Full discussion about possible consequences, including those a client might not foresee, is the first step in a process of seeking and receiving consent about any communication to third parties (6.1.a). The important point here is that the intended recipient of the original communication was the counsellor alone.

In addition, although a particular third party, such as a current or prospective employer, may be the intended recipient of the information passed on by the counsellor, there may be no guarantee that the information will remain with that person alone: in appointment processes, for example, such material is likely to be passed on to others involved in the selection process. Acting in accordance with the principle of informed consent (5.5), therefore, requires counsellors to advise clients of this possibility, including the potential risk that someone who becomes privy to the information may have some personal connection to the client. This risk is increased when a testimonial may be used in more than one job application or context (Winslade, 1998).

Futhermore, a request to allow the counsellor to share with one or more third parties what was initially written and intended as a personal communication within an established and trusting dyadic relationship, may risk leaving a client or former client feeling vulnerable, as if suddenly transported from the security and safety of a private room, onto the exposed space of an open stage. This request is made within the same relational context as seeking a testimonial might have occurred, as discussed above, influenced by the same distribution of power. The nature of this request is also qualitatively different from an invitation to a client to participate in a research project or to share a personal story in order to support and inspire others who are struggling with a particular challenge in life. In these situations, in which informed consent is necessarily sought, clients can benefit from knowing that they are contributing to the wider purpose of advancing knowledge and helping others (Winslade, 1998), while a testimonial benefits only the counsellor or the agency.

Rather than asking clients for permission to pass on personal communications to third parties, counsellors need to use other sources of information about their effectiveness, such as references from supervisors or from colleagues who have co-facilitated counselling processes. Seeking anonymous feedback in survey form from all clients about their experiences of counselling is a common part of counsellors' professional responsibility for monitoring their effectiveness as practitioners. If feedback from surveys and other sources is collated and presented in a way that protects client privacy, and in which no individual is personally identifiable, it can also form a valuable part of counsellors' professional portfolios, or of accountability processes for employing organisations, funding agencies, and other third parties, including counsellor education.

2.7 ETHICS FOR RESEARCH AND PUBLICATION

Sue Cornforth

The NZAC *Code of Ethics* (2002) encourages counsellors to engage in research in order to "inform and develop counselling practice" (11.1.a) and further advises that "counsellors should limit the demands of any research exercise to what can be justified in terms of benefit to individuals or the community" (11.1.b).

Research is thus embedded in ethical practice and can be viewed as a form of inquiry that invokes moral responsibility. Our responsibility is to engage in a reflexive process in which we keep abreast of current research and also consider the possibility of ourselves as researchers. We might think of ourselves as researching practice when on a day-to-day basis we reflect on our work with clients. When questions that arise in practice are taken further into systematic investigation, our research becomes formal. Research then enters a more public forum (11) where we evaluate and discuss the implications of private counselling practice. It is crucially important then, that we consider the ethical implications for all involved.

This section encourages practitioners to consider the possibilities of practice-based research based on ethical considerations. Questions we might ask when researching could include the following:

> What do I want to find out and why?
>
> What benefits do I, or my clients, or my whānau/community, or professional colleagues hope for?

> How does what I am interested in relate to what other counselling researchers have found?
>
> What can I learn from what's already been written?
>
> What new questions come out of this reading?
>
> Who else might it be appropriate to consult?
>
> How might what I have learned from reading be useful in my practice?
>
> Who might benefit from new knowledge that might be generated?
>
> What potential for harm should be considered?
>
> What might other researchers offer?
>
> Is it appropriate for me/us to actively engage in this research project?
>
> What are the ethical considerations?
>
> How can my inquiry be conducted and recounted in moral terms?

While research is serious and responsible practice, at the same time it can present exciting new opportunities for practitioners. Willig presents research as a sort of adventure – an exciting expedition into the land of new knowledge.

> It means venturing into new territory ...
>
> It's something that will develop me as a person ...
>
> [It's] an exploration involving new places, meeting new people and having new experiences ... (Willig, 2001, p. 1)

Here I offer a starting point in considering how ethics can act as a map or travel guide in a research expedition – to support you to map a preferred direction; to suggest that you do not undertake a potentially dangerous journey alone; in the hope that you might be well-prepared; and that your environmental footprints might be as light as possible.

It is an exciting time for such journeys as many of the old maps of research are being rewritten in order to deal with what Denzin and Lincoln (2005) refer to as "the triple crisis of representation, legitimation and praxis" (p. 19). This "crisis" has offered new ideas about how we represent others' experiences, how we evaluate research, and how we use research. It challenges old ideas about what constitutes knowledge, and about the ethics of knowledge production. In particular, feminist (for example Weedon, 1987), cultural (for example Smith, 1999) and postmodern (for example Scheurich, 1997) writers have suggested that traditional approaches to research have not always treated participants with respect.

However, whatever the theoretical position of the research, new knowledge is not something we create or find alone. Research claims must be comprehensible, useful and acceptable to others. McLeod (2003) described research as "a systematic process of critical inquiry leading to valid propositions and conclusions that are communicated to interested others" (p. 4). Research is thus about using and developing networks to discuss what is knowable. Crucially, research is about relationships and about being ethical in developing and enacting those relationships. Considering the ethics of relationship is familiar territory for counsellors. Coming to understand research as a practice of relational ethics was critical in her journey between counselling practice and research practice, suggested Crocket (2004, p. 67).

This section has as its focus consideration of the ethics of various research relationships: with the profession, research participants, other theorists, readers, any co-researchers and publishers. Each of these is considered in turn.

ETHICAL RELATIONSHIP WITH THE PROFESSION

Two core functions of NZAC are to "maintain standards of professional practice" and to protect the interests of clients (NZAC *Code of Ethics*, Introduction). How do we relate to these priorities as researchers?

Maintaining standards and proving efficacy

The NZAC *Code of Ethics* values research "in order to inform and develop counselling practice" (11.1.a) and encourages counsellors to maintain competent practice and engage in professional development (5.9). Researchers, and their "findings," and practitioners, with their practice-based knowledge, have opportunities to come together in dialogue. NZAC conferences and the *New Zealand Journal of Counselling* are two contexts for reciprocal sharing of knowledge within the profession. This research–practice relationship is one of the strengths of the counselling profession as increasingly we find ways to interweave these practices. Indeed, McLeod (2004) sees the type of small-scale, localised research projects that might emerge from some of these conversations as being crucial in influencing the direction of larger evidence-based, randomised control trials, at the same time as they benefit practice.

Research becomes increasingly important as more public funds are spent on counselling. Providers require demonstrated efficacy, whilst the current sociopolitical climate requires counsellors to define and defend their scopes of practice against those of other health professionals (Bond, 2004; Feltham, 2002). Research is now crucial to the future of the profession and we share a responsibility for this. However, in order not to research beyond the level of our competence (5.9.c), it seems important to think of research as a shared journey. Consultation is important and mentoring advice is available. Just as we contract and consult with supervisors for our counselling practice, so we should contract and consult with research supervisors for our research practice. As we make knowledge claims, as a product of research practice, the profession's credibility is at stake as well as our own.

Protecting the interests of clients

A key question is "for whose benefit is this research?" The NZAC *Code of Ethics* advises counsellors to "limit the demands of any research exercise to what can be justified in terms of benefit to individuals or the community" (11.1.b). Since a professional prerequisite is the primacy of the relationship with clients (2), we need to consider whether our project will ultimately benefit clients, directly or indirectly, or whether it arises out of the counsellor's personal material and offers no benefit to others. Exploring over-researched, sensitive themes can be voyeuristic, for example. Or, seeking clients' responses about the usefulness of therapy might be about bolstering self-confidence. However, there is much for us to learn about clients' views of therapy from studies that have been well constructed with the interest of clients to the fore (for example Manthei, 2006; Pettifer, 2003; Vallance, 2004). We might also think of seeking partnerships that support us to conduct research that values the interests of clients – through first consulting with the available literature, with a supervisor, perhaps with community groups, and in some instances with clients themselves.

Social justice and counselling values

McLeod (2003) writes "the ultimate moral justification for research is that it makes a contribution to the greater public good, by easing suffering or promoting truth" (p. 175). If one takes this definition, then engaging in research becomes one way of expressing core counselling values, particularly social justice (3.6). The sort of small-scale, practice-based studies that counsellors are likely to do allow us to express our commitment to "the equitable provision of counselling services to all individuals and social groups" (5.2.g). In them we hope to find what is meaningful for clients and their communities/whānau (5.2.e). Practice-based studies are therefore crucially important for several reasons. First, they are responsive to local needs and address those aspects of life and experiences that large, so-called evidence-based studies, often fail to even consider. Second, they allow us to foreground people who might otherwise be marginalised. Third, they allow us to continue to work with the human face of counselling partnership in collaborative projects. In Speedy's (2004) terms, these projects, in particular those narrative "research conversations" (p. 51) that include witness accounts, allow us to represent "a more peopled life" to the consumers of research. Speedy suggests that these peopled stories can make a strong impact on those who read them, and that therapists could collect a cumulative body of such practice-based "evidence" in order to influence the direction of policy makers (see also McLeod, 2004).

Ethical relationship with the profession requires:

- that we are up-to-date with current research;
- that we support the development of practice-based evidence;
- that research ultimately benefits our clients and their communities;
- that we uphold the values of the profession.

It also requires that we consider both research ethics and professional counselling ethics in any research we undertake as counsellors. Many of us will engage in research in the context of workplaces or academic institutions with ethical approval processes. We should honour these requirements along with our responsibilities to our professional *Code of Ethics*.

ETHICAL RELATIONSHIP WITH RESEARCH PARTICIPANTS

Although NZAC does not require its members to apply for ethical approval of research projects, the NZAC *Code of Ethics* alerts us to our responsibility to minimise risk (5.1): no-one should be disadvantaged by taking part in the research. The counselling values of respect (3.1), partnership (3.2), autonomy (3.3), responsible caring (3.4), and integrity (3.5) guide us to consider carefully the relationships we offer research participants. Current ethical thinking is much more aware of the relationships of power that exist between researchers and participants. Some of this thinking is founded on the work of feminist, cultural and anthropological studies that have made much more visible the responsibilities of researchers in relation with participants. The NZAC *Code of Ethics* indicates that we honour participants' contributions (11.7) and "avoid contributing to the marginalisation or objectification of people" (11.5.b). Our commitment to being trustworthy, offering participants clear and ongoing information about the research process, and ensuring our own competence as researchers are means by which we address the workings of power.

In working to build trusting, respectful research relationships that do no harm (4.2), a counselling researcher is responsible for the prevention and ongoing monitoring of any risk for participants. Ethical thinking requires that we thus anticipate what might pose possible harm for participants. I suggest that harm can occur in three main forms: outright trickery or misconduct, unwelcome surprises due to negligence and malpractice, and prejudice or failure to consider cultural safety (Cornforth, 2006).

Outright trickery

It is clear that any research in which the researcher benefits financially or sexually at the expense of the research participant, constitutes misconduct (5.12). However, taking up too much of participants' time, coercing consent from current clients, or using case studies containing sensitive material in order to make an impact as a researcher, could all also constitute misconduct. Our commitment to honesty (4.7) requires that we are open in our transactions and do not mislead participants or potential participants in any way.

Unwelcome surprises

Research can disturb participants' worlds in several ways. As a first step we need to provide sufficient information to allow potential participants to make informed choices (5.5) about whether or not to participate. The principle of informed consent involves us in providing clear and sufficient information, and also taking all possible steps to make declining as available an option for potential participants as we make consenting. Pathways for withdrawing should also be clear. Once the research is underway, we must manage and protect any potential vulnerability of participants, being sensitive in raising material that might re-traumatise, and being prepared for disclosures that threaten safety. We must describe for potential participants how we plan to store, access, use and destroy material in ways that protect privacy. We need to gain consent before publishing, or speaking about our research in any open or public context.

However, even with the best of intentions, surprises can occur, and it is a researcher's responsibility to manage these. Etherington (1996) suggested that counselling researchers may face particular problems by virtue of their specialist training in encouraging people to speak. She referred to "the tin-opener effect" (p. 346), referring to surprising disclosures about which we might need to consider our ethical responsibilities. She noted that the potential for harm, in this case, is not just for clients and third parties, but also for the counselling researcher: her physical safety and ongoing stress concerning the management of troubling disclosures. The possibility of negligence is mitigated not just by careful planning and forethought, but also by ongoing ethical thinking. Etherington's paper highlights the need for good, continued supervision in managing matters that continue to have a life beyond the research interview.

Intrusion of researcher bias

Various schools of thought about research understand differently the question of researcher bias. In the traditional scientist–practitioner model, participants can be harmed by taking part in a research project if they are exposed to researcher bias, that for example, involves a researcher "go[ing] in with a prejudice and coming out with a statistic" (Wild & Seber, 2000). In such a situation there is prejudice in the way information is gathered, and various strategies are called on towards producing trustworthy results (Kendall & Buckland, 1975).

In a social constructionist view, however, bias is understood as inevitable, in that neutral positions are not available. It is not being aware of, not declaring and not managing one's own interests and world view that are seen as problematic. Whatever the research methodology, the core values of counselling (3) demand that we build trustworthy relationships with participants and show respect for "individual and cultural difference" (4.1). When we impose our own unacknowledged world view on others we deny others' experience and values as well as the experience and values of those with whom they are associated. Relationships which are culturally unsafe result from lack of attention to this point. So, although bias affects the trustworthiness of our results (see below), it can also have a negative effect on participants by misrepresenting or negating their experience.

Research bias can be very damaging to members of minority groups, including women participants in particular. As many feminist and decolonising writers have noted, some bias is so deeply entrenched in our world view that it is easy to take for granted practices that other cultures or groups would find offensive. Constant attention to difference is thus important (for example Chantler & Smailes, 2004). One way of minimising this potential for harm is to declare our interests from the outset and thus avoid what Haraway (1988) calls "the god trick," or the assumption of universal knowledge. Another is to take the position of co-researchers with participants, working like "detectives together" (Speedy, 2004, p. 47) to negotiate new meanings. Another is to continually discuss our work with others – supervisors, ethics committees, cultural advisors – to ensure that we do not work beyond the limits of our competence. A further check is to build in reflexive processes that include opportunities for participants to comment on findings or withdraw their contribution up to a set time.

Ethical relationship with research participants requires, amongst other considerations:

- declaring our interests and position at the outset;
- ensuring that the researcher does not benefit at the expense of the participants;
- presenting sufficient information to ensure that fully informed consent is possible;
- thorough and ongoing assessment of risk;
- opportunity for participants to comment on, and to withdraw their contributions with a clearly specified end point;
- protection of participants' privacy;
- particular consideration given to difference and the possibility of gender, cultural and other forms of bias.

ETHICAL RELATIONSHIP WITH OTHER THEORISTS

As with any mihi,[1] researchers begin by acknowledging their academic whakapapa.[2] Introducing our research in this way acknowledges the work of others who have contributed to our topic, especially those who have

1 Greeting, tribute, in te reo Māori.

2 Ancestral and tribal affiliation, in te reo Māori.

influenced our thinking, and to frame more questions. With any mihi, as when working with clients, we must be scrupulous about the language we use in representing others. The same values of respect and careful responsibility (3) apply. The American Psychological Association (APA) citation and referencing format is designed to help us acknowledge and represent accurately the work of others.

The NZAC *Code of Ethics* offers an opportunity to go beyond the idea of critique as antagonistic (Sterba, 2001) – that is "critical thinking" being equated with adverse personal criticism – in offering the principles of partnership and respect (3) to guide the way in which we engage with other theorists.

Ethical relationship with other theorists requires:

- an accurate representation of their work;
- the acknowledgement of other relevant work;
- a generous and respectful tone, including when offering critique.

ETHICAL RELATIONSHIP WITH READERS

When presenting research it is important to keep in mind the audiences for whom we are writing. For example, practitioners are busy people and want value for time spent reading. Again, honesty and trustworthiness (4.7, 7.1.a) underpin the "fair and accurate" (11.8.a) reporting of results. In a counselling context the relevance of a study might be judged by its potential to make a connection with the reader's experience and its potential application to other practice-based knowledge. In this view reliability is informed by an ethic of social justice. It serves the moral function of research that "makes a contribution to the greater public good" (McLeod, 2003, p. 175) and invites others to participate in the research community. Inclusion is a particular strength of feminist and narrative inquiry (for example, Crocket et al., 2009; Speedy, 2004).

A further consideration relates to the intended audience of a research report. Will our reporting further the NZAC values of partnership and social justice, or is our focus primarily on meeting providers' needs to manage budgets, for example? In writing research reports we should be explicit about our purpose and our audience.

Our research reports should be transparent in reporting messiness and complexity (Bond, 2004, p. 15), problems and difficulties encountered, thus enacting the core value of integrity (3.5). Researchers do not need to present themselves as experts, but rather as fellow travellers advising others of difficult terrain.

Ethical relationship with readers thus requires:

- honesty and trustworthiness;
- consideration of audience and how the research may be used by others;
- a commitment to transparency.

ETHICAL RELATIONSHIP WITH CO-RESEARCHERS

The core value of partnership calls us to see beyond the idea of research as the achievement of an individual. At the least we should take account of relations of power with others. We should, for example, fully acknowledge co-researchers and other contributors (11.7.a). There are, as well, exciting possibilities in co-research that take us into what Denzin and Lincoln (2005) call "performing social justice" (p. 1124). These editors of the seminal text in qualitative research note an increasing range of research practices which open possibilities for a "rising tide of voices ... of the formerly disenfranchised" (p. 1115). In this way, research becomes, in itself, an ethical prerequisite.

Ethical relationship with co-researchers thus requires:

- acknowledgement of all contributions;
- openness to new forms of research;
- consideration of relations of power in our collaborations with others;
- commitment to research as an ethical practice.

ETHICAL RELATIONSHIP WITH PUBLISHERS

Finally, we have a responsibility to assist the effective communication of research through its publication. Research reports should include information about ethical considerations involved in the project. Crucially, material must not have been published before and material should be submitted to only one journal at a time. Book proposals, however, may be sent to more than one publisher at a time.

IN CONCLUSION

I have suggested that ethical research depends on the relationships we build with the profession, other theorists, research participants, readers, co-researchers and publishers. In this view, research extends counsellors' existing strengths. Lincoln and Denzin (2005) describe the future of research as "terra incognita to be explored" (p. 1115). I suggest that counselling ethics help us in preparing a chart for that exciting exploration.

Acknowledgement

I would like to acknowledge the generous support, experience and valuable advice of both Kathie Crocket and Bob Manthei in developing this chapter.

PART 3

SOME PRAGMATICS FOR PRACTICE

Following an overview about notes by Eric Medcalf, Carol White offers a companion-piece on notes. We use companion pieces at times in this book, on the basis that – as Jim Depree writes of his hopes for his companion-piece on even-handedness (see Part 3, Section 5) – perspectives taken together can add to the "depth perception" available to readers. (Eds.)

3.1
A FEW NOTES ABOUT NOTES

Eric Medcalf

Counsellors write up their work for a wide range of reasons: to record client information and significant events, to aid recall of progress, and to record interventions. Notes are written with a range of potential readers in mind – colleagues, supervisors, clients themselves and in some circumstances funders, employers, insurers and courts of law. This section is intended to promote thought, offer guidelines, cite law, and bring into awareness some of the traps into which, as counsellors, we may unwittingly fall.

The NZAC *Code of Ethics* provides guidelines for the ethical collection and disclosure of information relating to work with clients. This Code sits against a wider background of agency (including school) policies, and New Zealand law: statutes, regulations and codes. The law is rarely simple and its variety and complexity frequently require untangling. Just working out who is and who is not a "counsellor" can be complex. Counsellors who do not consider that they are involved in the business of "health" (for example, careers counsellors) are less constrained, as most of the legislation relates to counsellors who provide services which promote, maintain or develop good psychological health, whether they work in private practice or in statutory or non-profit organisations. Counsellors working in statutory settings are subject to additional law relating to "official information", to which counsellors in private practice or community agencies are not, unless information provided by them is held by a government agency (see below).

WHY KEEP NOTES?

Most of us are not blessed with perfect recall. Counsellors thus benefit from notes that help remember client details, assessments, interventions and plans, and aid reflections on both the counsellor's and the client's processes. Notes that benefit the counsellor should also benefit their clients. Counsellors should write notes with awareness of who else may read them in order to meet both professional and legal requirements.

The NZAC *Code of Ethics* states:

> Counsellors shall maintain records in sufficient detail to track the sequence and nature of professional services provided. Such records shall be maintained in a manner consistent with ethical practice taking into account statutory, regulatory, agency or institutional requirements (2002, 5.7.a).

New Zealand law has much to say about the collection of information, its storage and the limits of confidentiality. The Privacy Act 1993 has most relevance to *all* counsellors, with the Health Information Privacy Code (HIPC) and the Health (Retention of Health Information) Regulations 1996 applying in situations where counsellors are involved in providing "health and disability services." Which counsellors are governed by this particular regulatory environment is a matter of some debate, not unrelated to the current issue of occupational registration under the Health Practitioners Competence Assurance Act 2006. Debate on the statutory registration of counselling (Cornforth, 2006; Manthei, 2008; New Zealand Association of Counsellors, 2008) contains methodological and political arguments about the professional position of counselling in relation to mainstream health services and the so-called medical model. Counsellors working from other perspectives may not wish to align themselves with this position and might thus eschew the label of "health professional." Whether this is sufficient to absolve them from legal responsibilities related to reporting could only be tested by legal challenge. It can be noted that the HIPC comes down firmly by making specific reference to counsellors approved by the Accident Compensation and Rehabilitation Corporation as under its jurisdiction, with the obvious implication that counselling people who have what the Accident Compensation Commission calls a "mental injury" constitutes a health and disability service, and the counsellor is a health professional (Accident Compensation Act 2001).

The HIPC states that health information must not be collected by any health agency unless:

a. the information is collected for a lawful purpose connected with the function or activity of the health agency, and

b. collection of that information is necessary for that purpose.

Counsellors, whether working on their own, in a group, or in a public organisation are, according to the Privacy Act 1993 (Part 1 (2) "Interpretation"), "agencies."

The law says that a counsellor must inform clients that they are making notes (HIPC, Rule 3), and the notes must be stored securely so as to protect against loss or misuse, including unauthorised modification or disclosure (HIPC, Rule 5).

It is good practice for a counsellor to discuss the existence of notes at the commencement of the counselling and to obtain written consents on their appropriate disclosure. However, counsellors should bear in mind that the beginning process is when clients are most vulnerable, and the balance of power is most skewed in favour of the counsellor. Revisiting consents later on in the work, and especially when disclosure is considered, is respectful.

TYPES OF NOTES

The NZAC *Code of Ethics* uses the term "documentation" to include:

> ... all material about the client or about the counselling, recorded in any form (electronic, audio, visual and text). Documentation includes material collected for the purposes of: enhancing counselling practice; and meeting the requirements of research, accountability, appraisal, audit and evaluation. (2002, 5.7)

This is a wide definition and succinctly describes the types of documentation and the variety of purposes for which notes and reports may be written.

PERSONAL JOURNALS

It can be argued that some notes, especially those kept to "enhance practice," may not be subject to the same legal strictures as those which are specifically related to a particular client. A personal journal that is kept as a record of thoughts, conjectures, and reflections on the counsellor's own process may be a very useful parallel to their professional work, but because it is more to do with the counsellor than the client it can remain personal. If a counsellor chooses to write about his or her emotional and intellectual reactions to a client, including reflections and suppositions, these materials can be considered part of the counsellor's process and subject to *that person's* rights to privacy in situations where a client seeks access. They may, however, remain accessible in situations where proof of reflection, or discussion in supervision, is required, for example in the case of a formal complaint.

However, if a counsellor writes specifically about a client and the content of the sessions, then what is recorded, whether in a journal or not, will still form part of the record and be subject to the law on case records. It follows therefore that a personal journal may still be subject to a Privacy Act request. Such a request can be contested by a counsellor.

In any case a journal is still "documentation" and subject to the NZAC *Code of Ethics*. Notes about the counsellor's process may be kept with client notes, but the counsellor would be well advised to have them in a form that can be removed in situations where the client requests access. In other situations, such as a court order for access to the client's file, these notes would be seen as part of the file, with removal subject to legal sanction by the court. Generally, therefore, it could be argued that it is better to keep journal notes separate form client records.

ACCOUNTABILITY, APPRAISAL AND EVALUATION

As professionals, counsellors are accountable to their clients, their professional peers and, in certain circumstances, employers and third-party funders, for the quality of their professional work. Documentation must provide *sufficient* evidence of this so that, in the case of legal or ethical scrutiny, professionalism can be defended to peers or to the courts. Thus there must be evidence of thorough consideration of the issues brought by each client, of ethical behaviour, of planned work, its progress and outcomes.

There must also be sufficient recording of issues significant to the work, such as disclosures of abuse or other life events, how they have been made, and a clear exposition of the consequences for the client. This recording should enable another person to see the basis for the work being undertaken, and the justification for the approaches used. There must also be clear pointers to progress being made by the client, both in their self-report and in the counsellor's own observations in the session. The form of such notes will depend on the practice preferences of a particular counsellor. For example, notes may also include the use of structured self-report questionnaires, such as a trauma questionnaire, or depression inventory, scores on which might indicate change in the client's intrapsychic and social functioning. Similarly, notes are likely to record events such as new relationships, employment and changes in living situation.

HOW LONG DO I HAVE TO KEEP MY NOTES?

It is the opinion of the Ministry of Health that counsellors and psychotherapists are "providers" under the Health (Retention of Health Information) Regulations 1996. Providers of health services have to keep notes for a minimum 10-year period (Section 6.1). Failure to do so may leave counsellors liable to legal penalty. Section 11 of the Health (Retention of Health Information) Regulations 1996 states:

> Offence (1) Every provider commits an offence who fails, without reasonable excuse, to comply with regulation (6.1) of these regulations.
>
> (2) Every provider who commits an offence against subclause (1) of this regulation is liable on summary conviction to a fine not exceeding $500.

The issue of whether or not you are a provider under these regulations is, as I have previously suggested, a matter of some debate. Ludbrook (2003), while inaccurately naming these regulations and stating seven years, not 10, errs on the side of counsellors *not* being health providers. He differentiates between "general counsellors" and those who provide a health service. I would differ on this and suggest that *most* counsellors are in the business of providing a health service and are therefore subject to these regulations.

WHO HAS A RIGHT OF ACCESS TO NOTES, AND WHEN?

1. The Client

> The Health Information Privacy Code 1994 states: Where a health agency holds health information in such a way that it can be readily retrieved, the individual concerned shall be entitled:
>
> a. to obtain from the agency confirmation of whether or not the agency holds such personal information, and,
>
> b. to have access to that information (Principle 6).

However, there are situations where a counsellor may legitimately refuse to give a client access to the notes about them, in full or in part. These include situations where

> ... The disclosure of the information (being information that relates to the physical or mental health of the individual who requested it) would be likely to prejudice the physical or mental health of that individual.

> Privacy Act Part IV 29 (1) (c)(ii). Other examples can be viewed in the Privacy Act and its Code.

If access is refused, the counsellor may be challenged by a complaint to the Privacy Commissioner, so it is important that there are good records of decision-making processes, including when advice has been sought, and from whom.

Notes may also contain information that has been obtained from or about people other than the client. The client has no automatic right of access to these just because they are in the file, unless, of course, what has been said is about the client. An example would be copies of letters which refer to more than one person, including other family members, or notes of contact from third parties who may not want their identity to be revealed to the client. In this case that information should be extracted from the file, or deleted from a copy, so that the others' rights to privacy are not breached.

2. *Parents*

This is an area of some confusion, involving questions such as the child's competence to give informed consent, their rights to privacy, and the sheer practicality of parents, at times, needing to know. An example of the latter is parents' rights of access to their children's vaccination records. However, parents do not have an *automatic* right of access to information about their child. Under the HIPC a parent has right of access to information about their child, if under 16, but the Privacy Act treats children as autonomous individuals.

In considering this matter the New Zealand Mental Health Commission (2006) says:

> ... if an agency considers disclosure is not in the service user's best interests, perhaps because of family dynamics or because of potential harm to the therapeutic relationship, the family may be advised that a decision not to disclose has been made on clinical grounds. This may apply even when the service user is a child and the person requesting the information is their parent or legal guardian, as parents and/or guardians do not have an automatic right of access to their children's medical records. In the case of the very young there would seldom be reason to withhold the information from a parent or legal guardian, but circumstances, such as suspicion of abuse, may arise that render it necessary.

The situation can become more complex in cases where parents are separated and/or in conflict. Perhaps the above guidelines against unsafe disclosure would best be adhered to in situations where one or other parent seeks information from a counsellor. Consultation is recommended in such situations.

3. Funding agencies

A counsellor's client may give permission for notes and reports to be made available to whomever they wish, including bodies such as ACC, who may fund all or part of the counselling. They also have a right to check accuracy and to correct notes (HIPC Rules 6–8). The NZAC *Code of Ethics* states that: "Counsellors shall obtain informed consent from clients when writing reports for third parties" (2002, 5.7.b). It may be argued that clients, in signing the ACC claim form, are giving that permission. Counsellors would be wise to gain a separate permission from the client to disclose information about them to a funder in the same way that permission would be obtained to communicate with a GP or psychiatrist. Permission should be in writing.

Any permission from a client may have limitations attached – such as "*this* information, but not *that*" – and the permission may be rescinded at any time. Where there is third-party funding, the first ethical responsibility is to the client and if a client forbids the counsellor from providing information, the counsellor cannot go against that client's will unless forced to by a court of law. If a funder threatens to withdraw funding in the absence of permission then this decision may have to be challenged. The client may have to seek a formal review of that decision and be prepared to take legal action in order to retain the funding of their treatment.

The means by which clients have access to counselling notes may be varied. They might just wish to see them – a process helped by the presence of the counsellor or other support person. Others may wish to have photocopies of the notes. In this situation it is good practice to go over the notes first with the client. Where the notes and/or reports are held by a third party, then clients have a right to these. Clients occasionally ask for copies of their ACC files, for example. Counsellors or other agencies providing hard copy should advise the client of any risks attached, especially if the client then hands those notes over to someone else. In cases of prosecution, any evidence handed to the police is discoverable to a defendant's legal counsel, who may potentially use information to discredit the client.

Statutory agencies are subject to the Official Information Act which, like the Privacy Act, gives people rights to view and correct, if necessary, any information held about them by these agencies.

4. Employers

If the counsellor is employed in a school, university or community agency, for example, then legally the notes are the employer's property and it is that employer's responsibility to meet the demands of the law in relation to security, storage and confidentiality. Any personal journal, however, might be seen as *the counsellor's* property. Counsellors should work with agencies to develop appropriate policies and practices regarding records and notes. Often a counsellor may be the only representative of the profession in the agency, for example in a school, and should advocate that ethical and legal standards are upheld by their employer, especially regarding the storage and disclosure of records.

5. NZAC

The NZAC *Code of Ethics* provides for counsellors' notes to be available to the Ethics Committee in situations where a complaint is being investigated. Experience of handling complaints is that notes can sometimes be very useful, especially when they record out-of-session contacts such as telephone calls, and when they contain evidence of full reflection and ethical consideration.

6. Courts of Law

A counsellor may be required to present their notes in evidence in cases before a court. Sometimes this might be to support a client who is giving evidence in a situation of abuse. If this is with the informed consent of the client, there is no problem. A counsellor might, however, be requested by a defence counsel to present notes against a complainant (the client) in such a prosecution. An example might be a survivor of childhood sexual abuse who at some time worked as a sex worker. Despite legalisation of prostitution, a huge stigma continues to attach to women in the industry. Such information held in a file may be used to discredit the client's reputation in the eyes of a jury.

Counsellors' notes are not subject to legal privilege, but attempts by parties in legal action to gain access to notes should be defended against, and counsellors should obtain legal support in order to be heard by the Court. In order to resist such "fishing expeditions" courts may order the notes to be available in the first instance to the judge, who may then decide what, if any, information should be made available. See Part 5 for further discussion on legal aspects.

IF IN DOUBT

Often the law and ethical codes do not provide a definitive answer. Counsellors will benefit from open discussion of these issues with supervisors, peers and professional associations.

3.2 MORE NOTES ABOUT NOTES

Carol White

This section should be read alongside the previous section on notes by Eric Medcalf. The perspective in this section comes out of my counselling experience in education settings – schools and tertiary institutions – where counsellors have not been seen as health professionals (Ludbrook, 2003) and so the regulations of the Health Information Privacy Code (HIPC, 1994) have been less defining, particularly with respect to retention of notes. However, whatever the setting, while written notes may currently be the most common form, *documentation* (NZAC, 2002, 5.7) applies to any form of record, such as drawings or counsellor appointment diaries and electronic recordings such as audiotape, disc, videotape, email, information posted on the internet, voicemail and text.

COUNSELLING NOTES: CONTENT AND PROCESS

Some counsellors make notes during a counselling session. Others regard this practice as intrusive and write up their notes immediately afterwards, while some write them at a later time. Whichever approach is used, some form of documentation of the work undertaken is required in order to meet professional obligations to clients and the profession. A client has the right to expect to be informed, as part of a respectful informed-consent process, about the way notes will be produced and how their confidentiality will be maintained. Clients also have a right to see what has been written about them. If a client has concerns about what is recorded, there may need to be careful negotiation, in the light of both professional responsibilities and the client's concerns. Sensitive matters may need particular care. On the other hand, especially when plans for change have been developed and monitored and progress has been clearly documented, some clients find that being given a copy of their notes is extremely motivating. Other clients may like to have a copy of their notes at the conclusion of their counselling, as a record of their ongoing personal development.

It should be kept in mind that there may be circumstances – such as when a matter is before the court, when a request is made under the Privacy Act (1993), or at an Ethics Hearing – when there may be a wider audience to notes than just the client and the counsellor. Care should be taken to anticipate what might happen if others identified in the records were to gain access to the counsellor's notes and to ask how those records might be received and used in another forum, such as a court. Ludbrook (2003) advised that statements that potentially incriminate a client in a criminal offence should not be included in notes.

It is important to consider what factual information should be recorded. In the event that a counsellor assesses that a client is at risk of serious self harm or harming others, both the risk and a plan to address these concerns need to be documented. If a client discloses abuse or violence, the recording of any allegations against others should be undertaken with care. My practice has been to remember, rather than record, the identity of the alleged perpetrator of abuse, using terms such as *family member* or *close relative.* Privacy principles apply to information that can be linked to another person: someone who is identifiable, even if they are not named, can expect to have the right to access personal information recorded about them. However, it is also possible that a counsellor might be asked for information that can be recalled: the form of the information does not matter. In some circumstances it will be accepted that there are good reasons for refusing a request for access to personal information: to protect another person's safety; risk of jeopardising a criminal investigation; or if disclosure would unjustifiably breach another person's privacy (Katrine Evans, Privacy Commission, personal communication 26 March, 2010, and 27 July 2010).

Other matters to record may include who is present for a session, key concerns of the client, any mental health issues, details of medication, and any contact made with others regarding the client. Records should also be kept of missed appointments and any follow-up telephone calls, along with copies of written communication to and from other sources, including other professionals. In my practice I endeavour to record accurately a client's own words, using speech marks to indicate these. I take care to record, for example, a client's perceptions of problems, metaphors they produce to describe their situation, and goals, agreements or contracts developed through the counselling process. The usefulness of notes for keeping track of a client's story is well accepted. What use a counsellor makes of the notes of a previous session needs to be carefully considered, however, in the context of what is relevant to the client as a subsequent session begins.

STORAGE AND RETENTION OF NOTES

The NZAC *Code of Ethics* states that "counsellors should take all reasonable steps to ensure that documentation remains retrievable as long as is professionally prudent or as is required by law" (NZAC, 2002). Policies and practices regarding the retention and destruction of notes will likely vary from situation to situation, depending on the legislation, regulations, and codes of practice and ethics relevant to that context. Principle 9 of the Privacy Act states that information should not be kept "longer than necessary," and goes further to say "an agency that holds personal information shall not keep that information for longer than is required for the purposes for which the information may lawfully be used." These statements are relevant in the context of tertiary and secondary education. If counselling has been completed and the matters addressed are unlikely to be the subject of any future request for disclosure, and the student is no longer enrolled so cannot access the counselling service, then the justification for keeping those notes is debatable. On the other hand, Ludbrook (2003) advised that when there is a possibility that the matters addressed in counselling could be relevant at a later date, as evidence in a court action for example, those notes need to be retained securely. My practice has been to review any such stored notes annually to determine whether sufficient time has elapsed for the notes to be appropriately shredded.

OWNERSHIP OF AND ACCESS TO NOTES

Counsellors are responsible for informing clients about policies and practices in their setting in terms of ownership of, and access to, notes. Counsellors should be active in contributing to the development of such policies and practices, and ensuring they do not compromise ethical responsibilities, while meeting organisational needs and conforming to legislative requirements. In agencies where audits are ongoing, counsellors should inform clients of the practices that ensure their confidentiality, while providing an audit trail. In situations where such preparation has not occurred, the counsellor should provide non-identifiable records that give only information outlining the work undertaken and outcomes achieved.

In other circumstances where a third party, such as a lawyer, the police, a parent, caregiver or someone from an agency, asks for access to notes, a counsellor should seek professional consultation and legal advice. Depending on their client base, counsellors may be well advised to be familiar with the following, in addition to the legislation identified in Eric Medcalf's previous section:

Children, Young Persons and their Families Act 1989
Children and Young Persons Act 2008
Contraception, Sterilisation and Abortion Act 1977
Mental Health Act 1992
New Zealand Public Health and Disability Act 2000.

NOTES AND SUPERVISION

A counsellor may wish to refer to counselling notes during supervision. In order to assist the counsellor to refine their practice, the counsellor and supervisor need to be able to talk freely about the work. Making reference to notes or other forms of documentation will provide an opportunity for further development of the counsellor's practice. Both counsellor and supervisor are responsible for documenting supervision and for the safe storage of these notes. Notes provide a means of monitoring practice and should reflect the core value of responsible caring.

3.3 SCHOOL COUNSELLORS: CLIENTS, COLLEAGUES AND CONFIDENTIALITY

Colin Hughes

INTRODUCTION

There are few issues that are more central to a counsellor's effectiveness and reputation in a school than confidentiality. Confidentiality lies at the heart of the client–counsellor relationship as a key component in the development of trust. Any breach of confidentiality can have devastating effects on the counsellor's reputation amongst students in a school (Hawkins & Monk, 1995) with the result that, if the counselling service no longer seems to offer a place where confidences are safe, students may be at increased risk of isolation and powerlessness.

The school environment presents counsellors with particular challenges that relate to client confidentiality in working with colleagues.

Challenges include:

a. the shared nature of pastoral care responsibility among a variety of staff members: school culture tends to locate the decision to share information about a student with teachers or other authority figures, while counselling culture primarily locates the decision with the student;

b. different cultural concepts of confidentiality, especially among Māori staff, and the obligation to partnership under the Treaty of Waitangi (NZAC, 2002);

c. a counsellor's responsibilities to an employer (the Board and Principal) and responsibilities to the counselling profession may not always be aligned;

d. ownership of, and access to, the counsellor's notes.

THE CULTURE OF OPEN COMMUNICATION ABOUT STUDENTS AND SHARED PASTORAL-CARE RESPONSIBILITIES

Most secondary schools in New Zealand have a pastoral team who share responsibility for the welfare of students. The team usually includes counsellors, form teachers and, depending on the structure of the pastoral care network, deans, tutors, house leaders, careers advisors, and a member of the senior management team. While the counsellor is seen as having a specialist role and in many cases a leadership role, often as Head of Department, Guidance, the team aspect of shared responsibility for pastoral care is typically emphasised. This team approach to the pastoral care of students is often part of a school culture which values open communication about students among staff. Indeed, most schools spend considerable time and effort in facilitating open communication about students, to ensure that teachers and caregivers have up-to-date, relevant information about the welfare, behaviour and achievements of students.

The general belief may be that better outcomes for the student will be achieved if everyone has as much information as possible. However, for students themselves, this all-encompassing gaze can be uncomfortable, positioning them in ways that reduce the possibility of good outcomes. For example, a teacher may express an opinion which leads to another colleague negatively prejudging the student, thus affecting the quality of the student's relationship with staff, their well-being within the school and their learning outcomes.

The counsellor is positioned uniquely, and sometimes uncomfortably, between being seen by staff as a good team player who participates in the sharing of information, and counselling culture which requires professional commitments around what, when, and how client information is shared. A counsellor can be tempted to adopt an overly self-protective stance when dealing with issues that are controversial or may take a client safety perspective by deciding unilaterally to provide information to a third party. However, I suggest that honouring the core value of client partnership does require at times, that the counsellor alone amongst school staff, carries the weight of a difficult decision, because this serves the client's best interests. A counsellor's own feelings, perhaps of a sense of aloneness in the face of weighty problems, combined with pressures from colleagues seeking information, offer invitations to break confidentiality inappropriately that should not be underestimated. On the other hand, an elevated attitude of professional self-sufficiency that refuses to disclose or refer is also inappropriate.

> A fundamental understanding needs to be established that the safeguarding of individual privacy does not preclude the establishment of effective communication processes nor does it preclude the sharing of essential information in an appropriate manner. (Agee, 1997)

For the school counsellor finding their way amongst these competing demands, there is a clear need for regular professional supervision where such issues can be addressed. The impact of not getting this balance right can be professionally and personally serious.

Practice example

A form teacher approaches the counsellor at interval to share her concerns about a student in her form class. She reports that she had noticed an incident where William lashed out with some expletives when a student accidentally bumped his desk while passing by, a reaction which the teacher thought was uncharacteristic. She speaks to William at the end of the period, only to get an angry mutter of "Sorry." She then speaks to William's other teachers, and they report a dramatic drop in his work effort and that he seems unhappy. It is at this point that she speaks to the counsellor, asking him to see William.

The counsellor agrees, gaining the teacher's permission to be identified as one of those who have concerns. Subsequently William reveals to the counsellor that his mother, who parents her children alone, has been diagnosed with breast cancer. William has two younger sisters, neither of whom is aware of their mother's condition. William, who has been sworn to secrecy by his mother, checks with the counsellor that nothing he has said about his mother's condition will be repeated to others. The counsellor gives that assurance, and explores with William what might be most helpful to him for his teachers to know. After some discussion, William is happy for the counsellor to tell his teachers he is struggling with a greatly increased emotional load, and that he will have support from the counsellor during this time.

The next day the form teacher asks the counsellor whether he has "got to the bottom of the problem with William." The counsellor thanks the form teacher for her referral, saying William is facing a considerably increased emotional load and the referral was both timely and important. The counsellor explains that while William does not want to be quizzed by others, he is happy to continue to come to counselling for support, and that the form teacher could be of real help by reporting any continued concerns she might have regarding William's behaviour. The counsellor puts a similar message in writing to all of William's teachers.

Question to consider

In what ways does this example illustrate what Agee (1997) called that fundamental understanding of safeguarding individual privacy while not precluding effective and essential information in an appropriate manner?

Critical actions the counsellor took included:

- gaining the form teacher's permission to tell William of her concern;
- negotiating with William what the counsellor might appropriately tell teachers;
- acknowledging to the form teacher the value of the referral, and inviting contact about any continuing concerns;
- providing general information, including William's wish not to be quizzed, and that he was to continue to come to counselling;
- contacting other teachers with the negotiated information.

The counsellor also assured William that he would keep confidence about his mother's diagnosis. This was in addition to the general statement made at the beginning of counselling, informing William about confidentiality and the situations in which it did not apply.

MĀORI VIEWS OF CONFIDENTIALITY AND TREATY PARTNERSHIP OBLIGATIONS

The Treaty of Waitangi, and Māori as tāngata whenua, are given specific acknowledgement in the introduction to the NZAC *Code of Ethics:*

> Counsellors shall seek to be informed about the meaning and implications of the Treaty of Waitangi for their work. They shall

> understand the principles of protection, participation and partnership with Maori. (2002)

In New Zealand schools, partnership is given expression in a variety of ways, including in pastoral networks. Whānau concepts of organisation, with their philosophy of extended family and shared responsibility for each other, and the appointment of staff such as kaitiaki, whaea and kaumātua, are particular expressions of this partnership. These staff and systems of care bring an emphasis to confidentiality that often contrasts with a more individualistic Western tradition. Again, counsellors might meet competing expectations about the sharing of information, and have to work their way through competing ethical principles.

PRACTICE EXAMPLE

In response to the scenario of two fourteen-year-old girls wanting permission to have time off school to visit a Family Planning Clinic for a morning-after pill, Hawkins and Monk (1995) reported that Māori parents were unanimous that parents must be informed. This unanimity seemed to arise from two factors: the specific situation itself and the more general idea that the concept of client goes beyond that of just the individual to include the whānau. It was also made clear by a Māori parent: "The client to me is extended as far as Māori people go – the child – the parents need to know. So it is not just the child who is coming for counselling. Everyone else has to be drawn in, I think" (Hawkins & Monk, 1995, p. 5).

My 25 years of experience working in schools with very significant Māori student populations, and with many Māori teachers, suggests that the sentiments expressed by these parents would, mostly, be endorsed. A counsellor, for their part, is charged by the NZAC *Code of Ethics* to:

a. take account of their own cultural identity and biases and seek to limit any harmful impact of these in their work with clients (5.2.a);

b. work towards bi-cultural competence (5.2.b);

c. learn about and take account of the diverse cultural contexts and practices of the clients with whom they work (5.2.c);

d. seek cultural consultation to support their work (9.1.d).

In more general terms the NZAC *Code of Ethics* makes clear that its core values and ethical principles embrace both an individual and social dimension. For example, the first core value, "respect for human dignity," is reflected in the first ethical principle of acting "with care and respect for individual and cultural differences and the diversity of human experience."

In a discussion of the meaning of partnership around the NZAC *Code of Ethics* the question was asked, "Is partnership in the core values meant to refer to Treaty partnership? If not, partnership with whom?" The response was offered:

> It does refer to the principle of partnership in the Treaty. But we also want to say something here about all counselling relationships, not just those with Maori. The idea is that counselling relationships should not be exercises in colonisation. Counselling should always be a collaborative process in which at least two people make a full contribution, that is a partnership. (Winslade, 2002, p. 20)

Counselling therefore is first and foremost about a culture of partnership, regardless of the client's gender, race or age. That partnership relies on sensitive and accurate listening by a counsellor, informed by relevant cultural knowledge.

While offering guidelines, the *Code of Ethics* does not resolve philosophical questions about culturally constructed meaning. I refer to questions such as:

- who the client is;
- whether autonomy is to be interpreted primarily individually or collectively;
- whether partnership is primarily with the client, or would normally include others.

I suggest, however, that what is abundantly clear is that counsellors shall take into account both the individual and the cultural context. Some questions counsellors may find useful to consider are:

a. How might we as counsellors explore with clients the matter of confidentiality and their sense of cultural context?

b. In what ways can the counsellor mediate clients' fears around this matter?

c. How can these matters be explored with a client, without transferring pressure the counsellor might be feeling from other staff to persuade the client to adopt their position, regarding confidentiality?

d. How might we support and enable clients to identify and consider the perspectives of others who are significant in their lives, and how might we help clients to access support from within their own networks of family, whānau and friends?

e. What steps can the counsellor take to demonstrate to Māori staff members, especially those who have pastoral roles within the school, the counsellor's bi-cultural awareness on these issues and educate them on professional obligations around confidentiality?

It is the counsellor's responsibility to help any client explore the issues and implications around confidentiality, including the cultural context. To do this well, counselling skills should be well-informed by cultural knowledges. At the same time, the principle of autonomy, a core value of counselling in the NZAC *Code of Ethics*, would suggest that any client has the freedom to act outside their cultural framework.

THE COUNSELLOR'S RESPONSIBILITY TO THEIR EMPLOYER (BOARD/PRINCIPAL) AND PROFESSION

From time to time tensions can arise between a Principal's desire that parents be kept informed of certain critical issues, such as a young person who wishes to terminate a pregnancy, and a counsellor's legal and ethical position that a young person has the right to confidentiality (Ludbrook, 2003, pp. 258–259). The School Guidance Counsellor Guidelines state that:

The counsellor can expect that the Principal:

- trusts them and their judgements, at least until proved otherwise;
- will understand that the counsellor is bound by ethical considerations unlike those of teachers and will make sure confidentiality and the issues around this are rehearsed together, before a crisis occurs (Post Primary Teachers' Association and New Zealand Association of Counsellors, 2010).

Resolution of such conflicts requires good communication and trusting relationships (NZAC, 2002), the building of which can add significant value to the service counsellors offer to clients.

How then does a counsellor go about building a healthy working relationship with the Principal and Board, while maintaining adherence to the NZAC *Code of Ethics*? Counsellors need to empathise with principals' concerns, while at the same time making sure principals also understand the ethical and legal responsibilities of counsellors. The School Guidance Counsellor Guidelines (Post Primary Teachers' Association and New Zealand Association of Counsellors, 2010) provide excellent reference material in this regard. The mutual respect and trust that underpins genuine regard for one another's roles and responsibilities develops as we foster our relationships over time, and goodwill, commitment and skill are necessary to maintain such relationships. Our skills in working cross-culturally can be valuable assets as we work, as members of counselling culture, with senior staff and Board members who operate from a managerial perspective.

In my experience, it is common for school counsellors to agree that, if they are in possession of information where there is a medium to high chance it could become public knowledge and so cause embarrassment to the school, the counsellor would inform the Principal of the issue in a manner which protected client confidentiality, but also gave the Principal some prior warning. In this way the Principal can be prepared to respond to potentially controversial issues affecting the school's relationship with the community, in ways that protect the student, counsellor and the school.

Practice example

A 15-year-old girl came to the counsellor because she thought she was pregnant. The counsellor arranged for her to see the sexual health nurse the next day. The sexual health nurse confirmed that the young woman was pregnant and referred her to a doctor. During this process the student continued seeing the counsellor. The counsellor worked with the student to explore how she might be supported to bring her parents into the picture, but the student remained adamant that she did not want her parents to know about her pregnancy, or anyone else apart from the health nurse and doctor, and her best friend who had accompanied her to counselling, The 15-year-old student was quite clear she wanted an abortion. The counsellor was aware that:

a. the majority of the Board would be critical of the fact that the counsellor was not informing the parents

b. there was a medium to high chance that this girl's pregnancy would become more widely known through the client's friend

c. the Principal, who has final responsibility for the management of the school, would receive a considerable amount of criticism if the girl proceeded with a termination and the school had not informed the parents of the girl's pregnancy, and if this information became publicly known.

On the basis of this knowledge, the counsellor made an appointment to see the Principal a week before the termination was scheduled. In that meeting the counsellor:

a. outlined the situation in general terms taking care not to reveal the identity of the student

b. spoke of her work with the student, including the exploration of the student's desire not to inform her parents, the pros and cons of her position, and how she could be supported if she did decide to tell her parents

c. told of the girl's response to that process and the continuing concerns the counsellor had, and the girl's final decision to go through with the termination without her parent's knowledge

d. explained that the counsellor had taken this work to supervision and assessed the situation with her supervisor, who had affirmed the counsellor's approach

e. outlined the involvement of the health nurse and doctor, who had met with the counsellor for a case conference, and had taken an unequivocal position on maintaining confidentiality

f. confirmed the legal position which states that a girl can consent to a termination at any age (Daly & Holden, 1986), and that consent must remain confidential, as the normal rules of confidentiality apply (Ludbrook, 2003, pp. 85–86). Furthermore, "it is sometimes said that counsellors can breach confidentiality to protect or promote the welfare of the child. There is no general legal principle to this effect" (Ludbrook, 2003, p. 93).

g. stressed that the burden of professional responsibility was being shared by three different professionals, and that the counselling, and related consultations, had been careful, thorough and professionally competent.

Such an approach reassured the Principal, although it did not solve all the ethical dilemmas for either the Principal or counsellor.

Questions for the counsellor to consider

a. Do you agree with the counsellor's meeting with the Principal in the manner described?

b. What else, if anything, could the counsellor have done?

c. What factors are key in building a trusting relationship between principal and counsellor, and maintaining it in such a situation as this?

OWNERSHIP OF AND ACCESS TO COUNSELLING RECORDS

While the sections on notes earlier in this volume also apply in schools, there are some additional points that should be made. With regard to access to notes, Ludbrook (2003) suggested that, "a school counsellor's records should be kept separate from the usual system of student records and access to those records should be restricted to school counsellors" (p. 206). Student clients also have the right to access their counselling records, and it is important that counsellors inform clients about those rights and the degree of confidentiality associated with those documents (NZAC, 2002, 5.7).

While the matter of confidentiality of counselling records seems fairly straightforward, there are a number of aspects that require continual monitoring in the school counselling context. Some questions to assist this monitoring include:

a. Is the statistical information the counsellor abstracts for Board and other reports sufficiently protective of client privacy?

b. Are counsellors' paper and electronic records secure, that is, available only to the counsellor?

c. Is access to the counsellor's message answer phone sufficiently protected from others?

d. Are systems for securing counselling appointments protective of students' privacy?

With regard to this last question, it is my experience that it is in this rather mundane day-to-day issue that client confidentiality and privacy are most often compromised. Sometimes this compromise arises from a systems fault, such as students having access to an appointment book where they write their names next to appointment slots, or when counsellors themselves collect students from a classroom. Sometimes the problem is with the physical facilities, such as a waiting room which is open to view from a main walkway. Sometimes it is a problem of staff education, such as when a note is sent to classroom requesting a student see the counsellor, and the teacher reads out the note rather than handing it to the student. The counsellor has an ongoing responsibility to monitor the confidentiality of the referral process and its impact on students.

CONCLUSION

The NZAC *Code of Ethics* is predominantly about client–counsellor relationships. Therefore, while it acknowledges cultural context and others' voices with legitimate and legal concern for the client (for example, parents), the NZAC *Code of Ethics* gives the client the privileged voice over that of all others, except the voice of the law, and when serious concerns for safety are present. A school counsellor's professional responsibility is to combine skills and knowledge of the therapeutic counselling process, thoughtful application of ethical guidelines in practice, cultural knowledge, and good relational skills to engender trust among staff, students and school community, in order to provide the best service possible. That trust and that best service are, paradoxically, created by both the appropriate withholding of information and the judicious disclosure of information.

Finally, some practical suggestions:

a. Know your *Code of Ethics*. Diary time at least twice a year to read it through. It is well worth the effort.

b. Have on hand *Counselling and the Law* by Ludbrook (2003), which contains the legal guidelines within which counselling operates in New Zealand.

c. Ensure that the boundaries and procedures around client confidentiality are well understood by each client.

d. Ensure members of your guidance network take part in professional development around ethical practice in relation to their guidance/pastoral function.

e. Develop a variety of ways – print, staff meetings, student assemblies, newsletters – to talk about your role, including your practice of confidentiality.

f. If possible, rehearse with the client what you will say when sharing information with a third party.

g. Develop an understanding between yourself and other staff about how you negotiate the sharing of information a student has disclosed to you.

h. Affirm with staff the value of both sharing information and maintaining confidentiality.

i. Establish with your Principal a relationship of trust based on a shared understanding of your differing roles, and how you will seek to support each other.

j. Refer to the School Guidance Counsellor guidelines as a useful resource.

k. Ensure the privacy and security of records, both paper and electronic.

l. Ensure that processes are in place to protect student privacy when appointments are made to see a counsellor.

m. Continue to keep consideration of ethical dilemmas visible in supervision, and by attending workshops.

3.4
EVEN-HANDEDNESS IN RELATIONSHIP COUNSELLING

Rhonda Pritchard

> When dealing with more than one party, counsellors should be even handed when responding to the needs, concerns and interests of each party. (NZAC *Code of Ethics* 5.11.c)

Most people seek counselling as individuals because they need help with a range of presenting issues such as depression, stress, low self-esteem, loss, grief or trauma. Many, including those with individual concerns, also seek help because they are troubled in their relationships: with partner, with children, with parents and other family members, sometimes with friends or with colleagues at work.

If clients come alone, we can easily perceive them as the victim of another's mistreatment or neglect. Sometimes this perception is justified. In such cases, the role of the counsellor is clear: to provide support for the client as they prepare to protest, negotiate or disengage. In this situation, the client is left in no doubt about our alliance with them.

Often the picture is more complex. Most relationship difficulties arise from a blend of factors and more than one party is contributing in some way to the difficulties. I find that most clients are open to reflecting on the part they play if they feel respected, supported and understood.

Not all relationship counselling involves intimate partners. Often people seek help to heal or improve relationships with their parents, their children or with other family members. It is in the area of intimate relationship counselling, however, that the ethical requirement to be even-handed poses the greatest challenge to us as counsellors, especially if one of the partners is contemplating separation, or if the couple have already moved apart.

COUNSELLING COUPLES

When both parties in a relationship seek counselling together, each is hoping and expecting to be validated. In an ideal world they are each prepared to accept some of the responsibility for difficulties and for change, although most come with the view that the other is at least half "to blame." Human beings are not equally skilled at relationships any more than they are equally skilled at music, sport or mathematics. Indeed, one party may be more powerful, more mature, more skilled, more sensitive than the other. Sometimes one partner has done more damage to the foundations of the relationship, undermining safety, trust or respect: by having an affair, by excessive and secret overspending, by being violent or abusive to the other, or because they have a drinking or substance-abuse problem. Relationship partners are rarely in perfect accord about the balance of responsibility for the difficulties.

In many instances couples come to counselling at a point when at least one party is disengaging from the relationship. Often one is seeking our help to persuade the other to stay, while the other is hoping we will help their partner accept that the relationship is over. In the case of a separating couple, each might be determined to claim a greater share of care of the children, and we are asked to facilitate a mutually satisfactory agreement. In these situations, we may simply not be able to meet both partners' needs or desires.

These inequalities or competing interests pose a challenge for us as counsellors. While we are expected to be "even-handed," it can seem like an impossible task.

In practice, relationship counselling is more often a matter of "siding" with each partner, but at different times. Hendrick (1995) explained it this way:

> Although it may appear that the couple therapist is not initially taking sides the therapist is really siding with the relationship. This does not mean that the counsellor never shows bias toward either partner; it simply means that the bias is directed fairly equally to both partners, insofar as that is possible. It is rare to find a relationship in which both partners cannot be supported – and confronted – by the therapist. (p. 6)

From an ethical standpoint the guideline of even-handedness is not absolute or the only priority, and must be weighed against other principles and guidelines such as safety, responsible caring, promoting social justice and not doing harm. There will sometimes be relationship situations where one partner – in heterosexual relationships usually, but not always, the woman – needs to be supported to disengage or escape, because there is violence or abuse, and the other partner's immediate desires or interests have to take second place. The offending party can be supported, however, to change their attitudes and behaviour in their own long-term interests. This may mean referring them to other sources of help.

In most cases, however, while it is certainly challenging to respond equally to unequal power, unequal contributions to the problems, and unequal abilities to resolve them, there are ways to relate to both parties and manage apparently contradictory needs.

HOW DO WE PUT EVEN-HANDEDNESS INTO PRACTICE?

The following are some practical guidelines.

1. Notice our own response to each partner:
   - Do we identify with one more than the other partner?
   - Do we feel more irritated/frustrated with one partner?
   - What are the barriers to rapport?
   - If we were seeing this client on their own what would we have to do to build a relationship with this person?
2. At the contracting phase, invite the partners to say if they feel we are not being even-handed.
3. Notice if one partner is being silent or is becoming agitated and ask something like: "Have I missed something?" "Is there something I need to understand?"
4. Make turn-taking overt. "I'll ask each of you ..."
5. If one partner describes the other in a blaming or critical way, or accuses them of doing more damage than the other, ask the "accused" if they see it that way? Do they think this is a fair description?
6. Intervene in situations where there are tension-raising behaviours, such as 100 percent statements, labelling, analysing, provocative comments, domination of one partner by the other, and so on.
7. Describe the problem in terms of each person's concerns, needs or contribution to the problem, and each person's contribution to the solution *in the same sentence.*

8. Find a way to create alliance with the partner who has done more serious damage than the other, perhaps saying something like: "I'm imagining this might not fit with your own ideals or values" or "I'm presuming you don't want to make your partner scared of you."

9. If the tension is very high or the blocks continue, consider separate appointments. This is in accord with the Core Values (NZAC *Code of Ethics)* of autonomy and personal integrity, and the ethical principles of not doing harm, and of promoting safety.

GUIDELINES FOR INTRODUCING/CONDUCTING INDIVIDUAL SESSIONS (WHEN THE COUPLE IS THE CLIENT)

Reasons for individual sessions

1. The couple are separating;

2. To explore individual concerns, such as identity, sexuality, individuation, insecurity, stress, depression, anxiety, destructive patterns of behaviour, and so on;

3. Tension and hostility are high;

4. The counsellor is having difficulty with engaging with each partner equally;

5. One partner is very compliant, quiet or withdrawn.

The process of changing from couple to individual sessions

1. Discuss the idea and the reasons with both clients, or if one phones to make an individual session, ensure that the other partner knows and what the focus of the session will be. The following explanation is a way to emphasise that the counselling is for the interests of both clients and an indication of the counsellor's commitment to being even-handed: "If you tell me anything that significantly affects the trust, goodwill, intimacy or commitment in your relationship, something you haven't told your partner, I will need to know you have told them yourself before I see you together again."

2. Clarify the purpose and focus of the individual work.

3. Expect and promote the disclosure to each other of what is significant to the relationship, and what may be creating barriers to intimacy and commitment – and encourage partners to disclose to each other at home, as well as in subsequent sessions.

4. Ask for disclosure of current or recent sexual affairs. It is important that the counsellor does not collude with any secrets that disadvantage or exclude one of the partners, remembering that the counsellor is ethically required to respond to "the needs, concerns and interests of each party" (5.11.c).

From individual to couple counselling

1. Consider the effect on the initial client of changing your role and prepare that person well, especially if the one-to-one counselling relationship has been longstanding;

2. Offer the other partner an individual session;

3. Affirm that both partners are now your clients.

Even-handedness is relevant when we are counselling individuals in respect of their relationships with others, or when we are counselling couples or families, or working with groups. It can become particularly important when we engage in multiple roles, that is, when we move from counselling one member of a couple to counselling the couple, or when we work in mediation between one group and another, in a situation where some parties have been our counselling clients and others have not.

3.5
EVEN-HANDEDNESS IN RELATIONSHIP COUNSELLING: A COMPANION PIECE

Jim Depree

My approach to counselling is to treat it as a particular kind of collaborative and ongoing process of "ethical problem-solving" (Bond, 2000). Counsellors are responsible for clarifying the ethical obligations, legal rights and agency policy which are necessary to produce an "informed consent conversation" (Fisher, 2009) that promotes safety, fairness and respect. Accordingly, I preface my couple counselling sessions with some additional statements such as these:

> My job is to support each of you to express your view in a way that is respectful, safe and fair, so that you can be in a position to appreciate and then follow your own good advice. Please let me know if you feel you are not being given a fair say, or if you think I am taking sides, or if you feel we're off on the wrong track, or if you have concerns that our conversation will make trouble for you after you leave this room. Please let me know if you have concerns about how counselling is going. I can see either of you on your own. If you meet with me by yourself, then the usual confidentiality requirements and exceptions still apply.

This preface also includes explaining the policies that pertain to their situation, such as the procedures that apply to Family Court clients.

I have found White's (1986) "appreciation of difference" exercise useful for creating the conditions for informed and just decision-making and consent in couple counselling. White suggested that developing understanding, appreciation and respect for each person's view produces a "binocular" exploration of the problem and possible solutions in the same way that a view from each of our eyes is necessary for depth perception (p. 11). This "binocular" approach, which develops each person's distinct view, also serves as an alternative to the potentially unjust practices of power that require one person to submit to the other person's view of the truth. Similarly, counsellors have a duty to position themselves so that they are not imposing their views and that clients are not under pressure to adopt the counsellor's views (NZAC, 2002, 5.2.a, 5.5).

To promote clients' autonomy and counselling teamwork in relation to clients' hopes, I check out their experiences of the counselling with the following kinds of questions:

> Are we talking about the things you had hoped to talk about? What effect is this conversation having on you and your relationship? Do you feel you are getting a fair say? Do you have some ideas about how to improve this conversation?

I aim to ask these kinds of questions at the half-way point of each session, at the conclusion of each session, and at any time when I sense that clients might experience discomfort with how things are going.

At the outset, I make explicit a basic requirement of even-handedness by stating that I will be keeping an eye on the time each person has to speak, that I will stop interruptions so that people will have time to develop their thoughts. However, as some couples have told me that at times it was helpful and reassuring to hear what their partner was thinking, even if that meant he or she talked more, I find that my monitoring of their speaking must not overrule the couple's informed feedback.

Nonetheless, the ethics of ensuring safety and promoting diversity and social justice require more than that each person has the opportunity to have an equal say. Social, cultural and economic changes in New Zealand have meant that what is considered fair and appropriate in relationships and family is often contested (Claiborne & Drewery, 2010). As Rhonda Pritchard notes in the previous section, each person has different relationship skills. People do not have the same access to words or stories that might accurately represent their experience, nor to experiences that support confidence in what they say and the development of the skills to say it. People have different experiences of being heard, depending on whether what they are saying, skilfully or not, is acceptable to the listeners and to society in general. People speaking from taken-for-granted positions are likely to be seen as being right, while people speaking from less dominant positions may be seen as mistaken, unreasonable, or oversensitive (Bird, 2004). For example, I remember a conversation where I asked that my wife be referred to as Ms Tania Depree on correspondence rather than Mrs Jim Depree. The response suggested that we were mistaken, and that I was weak and Tania was overbearing or oversensitive. These reactions persisted despite our skilful expressions of our wishes and the absence of any authority of the other party to decide how Tania should be addressed. While this form of positioning from over twenty years ago might seem obviously problematic now, I suggest that, given the rapid changes in society, it is not safe to take a position of authority based on our current taken-for-granted or treasured positions. Instead, we have an ethical duty to assist couples to explore safely what they are standing for, what they might consider fair, and what authority they might be invoking, as part of a respectful negotiation of their preferred solutions.

The prevalence of violence to women and children in New Zealand families (Fanslow & Robinson, 2004) means that a counsellor cannot assume counselling conversations are safe for the persons involved. An accurate awareness of the possibility of violence requires a counsellor to be mindful that the threat of violence may be silencing one of the parties, or that speaking honestly may have violent consequences or other forms of retribution.

Therefore, *prior* to the disclosure of risky information, I advise my clients that to safeguard their relationship we have a duty to explore the potential effects of honesty and openness. Where violence has occurred, I prefer to have at least one meeting with each party prior to joint couple counselling. These meetings involve identifying risks and strategies to promote safety. Such strategies might include agreed signals and procedures if someone is feeling unsafe, and ensuring that the parties have the opportunity to leave separately. I ask questions that establish that no harm is being done by the conversation and to investigate what we can do to make it safe to continue.

Furthermore, couples often speak in and on the terms of the problem that has brought them to counselling, and such conversations limit what it is possible to say and the solutions that are likely to be considered. For example, when one person has been subjected to sexual abuse, then the effects of this abuse might be presented as *the* problem. In this situation, the fact that one person does not want to have sex sometimes may be considered an effect of sexual abuse without consideration of her or his right to not have sex. Simply accepting a narrow definition of the problem denies the couple the opportunity to make informed decisions about how they can work together to create intimacy, and may recruit the couple into strategies to help one partner ignore her or his preferences and rights to say "no." Rather, even-handedness is produced through a binocular exploration that goes beyond the taken-for-granted terms with which the conversation began.

I suggest that ethical problem solving requires ongoing binocular exploration and review of both the content and process of counselling by the counsellor, *with* the clients, and with the support of a supervisor. I believe that when these conversations include an explicit focus on, and review of safety, helpfulness and fairness, then they satisfy the ethical principles of counselling. I suggest that this approach also increases the chances of successful outcomes in our diverse and changing world.

My hope is that my piece on couple counselling will stand alongside Rhonda's piece as an example of binocular vision, so that our perspectives taken together add to the depth perception of even-handedness in counselling couples.

3.6
MULTIPLE RELATIONSHIPS

Kathie Crocket

At the heart of negotiating multiple relationships and roles is counsellors' professional responsibility to safeguard counselling relationships for the work of counselling. Interconnections of kinship, friendship, acquaintanceship, and business relationships shape counsellors' ordinary everyday lives and professional practice, whatever communities they live in or belong to. For counsellors in smaller or more strongly connected communities – church; lesbian, gay, bi-sexual, trans-gender, and inter-sex (LGBTI); or rural, for example – professional relationships in the context of, or alongside, other forms of relatedness become both more likely and more complex. There is a particular New Zealand-ness to consider, too: the understanding that identity and health are produced by relational connections (Durie, 1999, 2001) has particular implications for how the central counselling value of responsible care is practised in Aotearoa. Joy Te Wiata writes of the benefits of relational connection earlier in this volume (Part 1, Section 2): she has also suggested that whakawhanaungatanga might be seen as a process of making clients "kin" for the time and purposes of therapy (personal communication, 4 May 2010).

This section of the book begins with a general discussion about negotiating ethical practice in multiple relationships and roles, before focusing in particular on pastoral counselling (Philip Culbertson), and counselling within LGBTI communities (Antony McFelin).

WHAT ARE MULTIPLE RELATIONSHIPS?

Multiple relationships occur when a counsellor has other kinds of relatedness beyond the counselling relationship, either directly or by association, with a client. The other relationship(s) might be formed before the counselling takes place, while counselling is ongoing, or after the counselling has ended. Multiple relationships may involve a professional relationship in the context of a non-professional relationship, or multiple professional roles with the same client, family, or community group (Cottone, 2005). Multiple roles occur, for example, when a school counsellor who has been counselling a young person whose parent is dying, then becomes that young person's advocate at a suspension meeting with a Board of Trustees committee, and subsequently a referee for a job application. Multiple relationships might come about through a counsellor's chosen action, or by chance. A school counsellor may knowingly engage in counselling with a colleague's son, or a counsellor in an agency may have met with a client over some time before learning that the client is a member of her partner's wider family. In order to safeguard the effectiveness and potential of the counselling relationship, or to avoid undermining the benefits of counselling that has already taken place, counsellors must pay particular attention to the potential for competing roles or responsibilities.

Potential difficulties with engaging in overlapping relationships, identified by early commentators such as Pope (1991), included: the possibility of divided loyalties with divergence of responsibilities and conflicts of interest; different role expectations associated with each kind of relationship and the potential for incompatible expectations on the part of clients; and the ways in which power relations are enacted in different situations. In navigating the complexities of overlapping relationships, both clients and counsellors may experience vulnerability, ranging from confusion to a sense of betrayal, when the expectations and power relations associated with one relationship, such as a collegial friendship, are taken into and thereby undermine a therapeutic relationship. There is potential for the quality of both forms of relationship, including goodwill, to be damaged.

While the term *dual relationships* has been commonly used, the term *multiple relationships* is generally preferred as more accurately representing the many complexities of overlapping relationships and roles. Cottone (2005) suggested that neither term be used, but rather that there should be a re-focus to discerning "detrimental therapist–client relationships" (p. 1) from potentially beneficial overlapping relationships. Others have argued that multiple relationships take place on a continuum from "destructive" to "therapeutic" (Moleski & Kiselica, 2005), and that the key distinction is between "boundary crossings" and "boundary violations" (Lazarus & Zur, 2002, p. xxvii).

NEGOTIATING COMPLEX RELATIONSHIPS

There is a growing body of literature focused on complexity (Lazarus & Zur, 2002; Zur, 2005a) rather than prohibition, on connectedness rather than professional distance, and on managing or navigating through these complexities in ways that strengthen, rather than undermine, counselling relationships. The focus turns then to a contextual, relational practice of ethics, particularly informed by understandings of the implications of professional power relations.

The power relation inherent in counselling produces a potential for harm to clients: by its nature the counselling relationship is not an equal one. Harm through inappropriate professional–personal relationship overlaps may occur through inattention, but tends to occur when a counsellor's self interest or other priorities obscure their responsibilities to counselling relationships – to their client and/or a client's family, and to the profession – and as a result some form of exploitation occurs. A lack of attention to these responsibilities is, of course, not likely to be in the counsellor's own professional interest; it carries potential for harm not only to clients or those connected to clients, but also to themselves, their family, and their career.

An example of self interest might be the actions of a counsellor who counsels a separating couple, and subsequently forms a friendship with one person in the couple, without regard for any ongoing professional responsibilities associated with the counselling role, to the other person. On the terms of the NZAC *Code of Ethics* (2002), counsellors are not barred from ever forming alternative forms of relationships with those who have been clients, but always carry the responsibility to avoid doing harm. In this subsequent friendship situation, there is the potential harm of undermining the benefits of the counselling, along with the possibility of bringing the profession into disrepute, through the appearance, at least, of favouring the party with whom the friendship has developed.

It is unfortunate that instances of professional violation can have the effect of reifying professional boundaries, and making any boundary crossing seem problematic, rather than potentially therapeutic. The negotiation of boundary crossings involves a high degree of astuteness and skill. These professional responsibilities are particularly relevant to counsellors who belong in communities connected by close ties of membership, or those that have limits to their membership, where overlapping relationships are likely to occur. For example, there is a literature that investigates the particular situation for LGBTI counsellors (Kessler & Waehler, 2005, for example); and for practitioners in rural communities (Campbell & Gordon, 2003; Mellow, 2005, for example); as well as for those in religious communities (Hill & Mamalakis, 2001).

IS THERE A DIFFERENCE BETWEEN A CLIENT AND A FORMER CLIENT?

This question applies to many kinds of relatedness, but has been considered particularly in terms of romantic or sexual relationships. Some North American codes of ethics have tried to distinguish between a client and an ex-client by prohibiting sexual relationships for a nominated time period beyond the end of the therapeutic relationship (Welfel, 2010), while the responsibility for demonstrating that there is no exploitation involved in any sexual relationship remains with the professional. At the same time, there is a strong strand of argument in the literature that a sexual relationship with a former client is never ethical, based on the opinion that there will always be elements of the therapeutic relationship present (see discussion in Mattison, Jayaratne & Croxton, 2002, for example). Others argue that the construction of a lifelong permanent state of clienthood is patronising, suggesting that a brief period of clienthood should not forever restrict a person to the category of client, as permanently occupying the category of "helpless and vulnerable" (Zur, 2005b).

The NZAC *Code of Ethics* (2002) does not offer a time limit in its prohibition of sexual or romantic relationships with clients: "Counsellors shall not engage in sexual or romantic activity with clients" (5.13.a); and "Counsellors shall not exploit the potential for intimacy made possible in the counselling relationship, even after the counselling has ended" (5.13.b). All ethical responsibilities to the original therapeutic relationship continue beyond some fixed time period. The question here is about *exploitation* of the potential for intimacy made possible through counselling. Clearly, any decision to enter a romantic or sexual relationship with a person who has been a client should be approached only with great caution, clear and robust consultation, and vigorous investigation of the implications and ethics of such actions. Such consultation should include, and go beyond, a counsellor's usual professional community. Where there is potential for harm in engaging through overlapping relationships, seeking wider perspectives eases the potential that those who care for us professionally see things too much on the same terms as we do.

MORE ON THE NZAC *CODE OF ETHICS* AND MULTIPLE RELATIONSHIPS

The matter of safeguarding the counselling relationship is woven into the NZAC *Code of Ethics* from beginning to end. Section 5 offers general guidelines about the counselling relationship, including guidance for making decisions where there is, or may be, an overlap between our professional and personal lives, or between professional roles. Clauses 5.11, Multiple Relationships; 5.12, Exploitation; and 5.13, Sexual Relationships with Clients are particularly relevant. These clauses call counsellors to think through relational actions outside counselling with those who are clients in counselling; and inside counselling, with those with whom counsellors have had, currently have, or might have, connections outside the counselling relationship. The call to assume "full responsibility for setting and monitoring the boundaries between a counselling and any other kind of relationship and for making such boundaries as clear as possible to the client" (5.11.a) is about safeguarding the counselling relationship for the professional tasks of counselling. Similarly, the prohibition of sexual relationships with clients (5.13.a), perhaps the most stark example of a detrimental multiple relationship, has as its central concern not doing harm, again safeguarding the counselling relationship for the work of counselling.

The NZAC *Code of Ethics* positions counsellors, supervisors and our professional communities to think through our responsibilities in the light of the values, ethical principles and guidelines it offers. While there are some calls for ethical codes to offer practitioners clearer rules or definitions (Mattison et al., 2002), most recent international literature argues that each situation requires a process of careful assessment in terms of general ethical principles, since it is impossible to legislate for every possibility. In the literature there are many models on offer for making such assessments (Hill & Mamalakis, 2001; Kessler & Waehler, 2005; Younggren & Gottlieb, 2004). This section draws on these models in its suggestions.

FINDING OUR WAYS FORWARD

Any situation in which there are complex multiple relationships calls for counsellors to be clear about their responsibilities, to notice and pay attention to questions arising and to attend to them with care. They should engage in rigorous consultation and discussion in supervision, consultation groups, staff teams and other appropriate professional situations. Rigorous consultation offers protection to clients and counsellors that warm reassurance might not. What follows are some possible areas for consultation to traverse, Code in hand, not because the Code offers blind rule-following, but because it offers the current wisdom from the professional association about the values that are integral to counselling practice, the principles by which those values are enacted and the guidelines to follow in these enactments. It offers further dialogic voices into complex discussions about complex situations.

The following should be considered in weighing up the appropriateness of various forms of multiple relationships.

(a) Relatedness before counselling begins

1. The nature of the already existent relationship(s);
2. The availability of other services for the person seeking counselling;
3. The possible effects, beneficial or problematic, on the already existent relationship(s), for the client and for the counsellor, or for others in the client's or counsellor's lives;
4. The understandings a counsellor's own theory of practice offers, and the contrasting understandings other theories of practice might offer;
5. Experience in negotiating one's way between counselling and other roles and relationships;
6. What the client wants from counselling and how they want to get there;
7. How the counselling has been proposed, and by whom;
8. The kind of professional support available to the counsellor while engaging in the counselling relationship.

Some questions for reflection and discussion

- How might it be different if the person requesting counselling is the fruit grower from whom you buy strawberries, or a kaumātua from your partner's marae, or the recently separated partner of another client?
- Does it make a difference if you are the only available ACC-approved counsellor in your rural area, or if the other gay counsellor to whom you hoped to refer this person has a long waiting list?

(b) Taking up other forms of relatedness during counselling

1. How this potential new relationship came about;
2. The possible effects, beneficial or problematic, this new form of relatedness might have on the counselling relationship;
3. Who this new form of relatedness serves;
4. What courses of action may offer alternatives to pursuing this other form of relationship;
5. The understandings a counsellor's own theory of practice offers, and the contrasting understandings other theories of practice might offer;
6. The nature of the client's concerns and the therapy;
7. The kind of professional support available to the counsellor while engaged in the counselling relationship.

There are also those circumstances where another form of relatedness is not chosen, but which a counsellor nonetheless has responsibility to manage – such as a school counsellor who is seeing a student who then trials for a sports team the counsellor coaches.

Some questions for reflection or discussion

- In what situations do you meet clients outside your counselling practice?
- Which of these situations is most difficult for you? Why?
- In what circumstances do you think it would be OK for a counsellor to meet with a client for lunch to honour the ending of a therapeutic relationship? Who should pay? Why?

(c) Taking up other forms of relatedness after counselling

1. The nature of the new form of relatedness to be taken up;
2. How the counselling came to an end;
3. What kinds of assurance, to do with the client, their whānau and the counsellor, would be necessary to determine that the counselling was finished, and that there would be no likelihood of any request for further counselling;
4. The focus of the counselling;
5. The duration of the counselling relationship.

Some questions for reflection and discussion

Julie, a school counsellor, supported Hinemoa, a student, through difficult times during Years 9 and 10 when Hinemoa's relationship with her mother and custodial parent, Maureen, was particularly turbulent. Hinemoa is now in Year 12. Would it be appropriate for Julie to join a waka ama team of which Hinemoa's mother is the leader? What considerations would be relevant?

SOME SUGGESTED ACTIONS, IN NO PARTICULAR ORDER, IN RESPECT OF RESPONSIBLE PRACTICE AND OVERLAPPING ROLES AND RELATIONSHIPS

1. Consider potential benefits and harms to individuals, families, communities, and the profession. Read. Consult the NZAC *Code of Ethics*. Follow up the references in this book and read more widely.
2. Discuss. Review thoroughly any decision to engage in relationships that overlap, and the ongoing counselling and/or relationship development, with a supervisor/consultant who is willing to be honest and rigorous in your shared investigation.
3. If that person agrees with you, ask another professional for whom you have respect who might bring a different perspective.
4. Record the processes of identifying a concern and thinking through your actions.
5. Consider if this is a situation when you, or you and your supervisor, might responsibly involve the client in discussion

of the complexities. In what other ways might the client's understandings become directly available to the considerations?

6. Notice, and think through honestly, what benefits there are for you, and others in your life, in the decision. And then, think it through again.
7. Notice, and think through, what costs there are or might be for your client, or their family, or others in their life, in the decision. And then, think it through again.
8. Notice the effects for you of the costs of making professional distinctions. Review these with another professional. Honour the ongoing professional discernments you make.
9. Imagine the actions you plan to take or have taken. Ask yourself if these actions fit with the story you have of yourself as a professional counsellor. Ask yourself whom you might invite to witness your telling of this story in ways that acknowledge the professional skills and wisdom you enact in your work with clients.

3.7
MANAGING COMPLEX RELATIONSHIPS IN PASTORAL AND CHURCH-BASED COUNSELLING

Philip Culbertson

A complex relationship exists when a lay or ordained pastor, or anyone responsible for the pastoral care of others, serves in the capacity of both counsellor and at least one other role with the same client. Frequently, the additional relationship is social, financial or professional, as well as concurrent with the responsibilities of direct pastoral care. Other forms of mental healthcare discourage or even forbid contact with clients outside the counselling room, but in pastoral work such restrictions are often unachievable. Yet complex relationships present repeated dilemmas that are, first and foremost, the responsibility of the counsellor to manage.

IDENTIFYING COMPLEX RELATIONSHIPS

Church-based work often assumes that one can be simultaneously a pastoral counsellor and "a friend in Christ." From the perspective of other mental health professions, this is a questionable assumption, but because the idea is rooted in the New Testament's portrait of Jesus (John 15), it often lurks silently within the church-based relationship. This automatically makes relationships complex, in that the counsellor carries a dual set of expectations. Consider these possible dual or multiple role relationships:

- A male pastor may be asked to counsel his female associate (or vice versa), possibly introducing complex issues of authority, gender and sexual attraction;

- A pastor may be asked to counsel a member of his own family, introducing complex issues of family dynamics and of confidentiality;
- A pastor may be asked to counsel someone who, in another capacity, has authority over the pastor's employment conditions, introducing complex issues of power and transparency;
- A pastor may be asked to see a child, possibly introducing complex issues of exploitation by an adult authority figure, and the vulnerability of young people;
- A pastor with one cultural identity may be asked to counsel a congregant with a different cultural identity, introducing complex issues of values and worldviews;
- A church-based counsellor may be asked to pastor two members from the same family in the congregation, about two different problems, introducing complex issues of safety and privacy;
- A pastor may seek counselling with a practitioner within her or his own church community;
- A lay counsellor may hear disturbing information about a member of the clergy team from a client/parishioner.

Every human being lives in the midst of complex relationships, especially in small or rural communities. The literature's consensus is that complex relationships are both rich and often ethically dangerous for those in church-based work (Claret, 2005; Haug, 1999; Miller & Atkinson, 1988; Parent, 2006; Syme, 2003). Managing multiple role relationships and preserving appropriate boundaries of confidentiality are arguably the greatest challenges for counsellors working in pastoral contexts. Given the complexities, it is critically important for church-based counsellors to be well educated in pastoral ethics; knowledgeable about legal and accountability restrictions on what they do; alert to power issues of culture, age, gender inequality, sexuality and so on; and actively supported by high-quality supervision.

PARTICULAR ISSUES IN PASTORAL ETHICS

Church-based counsellors may serve in inwardly turned communities – communities concerned with their self-preservation, and committed to a vision which may be at odds with that of the wider community.

This dynamic may encourage pastoral counsellors to make friends inside the church community where they serve, raising the issue of "predatory professionalism," that is, using the pastoral relationship to meet the counsellor's needs. Pastoral counsellors, as much as possible, are encouraged to form their friendships outside, rather than inside, the congregations where they work (Doehring, 1995).

Pastoral counsellors must observe absolute boundaries around sharing, in any other context, information obtained during pastoral counselling – apart from the standard exceptions to confidentiality that apply in any counselling setting (NZAC, 2002, 6.2). Such issues can be ethically and morally complex, and even contestable. In a situation of doubt concerning our responsibility to observe professional ethics in a situation, for example where we do not wish to be complicit in some kind of harm, our supervisor should always be consulted. Otherwise, nothing about those we counsel should be disclosed without their express permission. What may seem inconsequential to the counsellor may be deeply held by the client. Appropriate boundaries may differ from counsellor to client. A pastor's seemingly innocuous reference to someone else can easily become grounds for breach of trust allegations. No one, including the pastor's spouse, the person's family members, other church workers, and members of the congregation, should be privy to information disclosed by a client in a counselling session.

Many New Zealand churches require supervision for clergy, and best practice suggests that this supervisor should be outside the immediate faith community. I believe that non-ordained pastoral counsellors should also engage in regular professional supervision. Supervision not only supports the counsellor in ethical and legal safety; it also functions as an invaluable form of ongoing training. Minimally, a pastoral counsellor should engage in one hour of clinical supervision for every 20 hours of counselling; less-experienced counsellors should have supervision more often (Culbertson, 2000).

Those who seek counselling in a church setting may not understand the difference between pastoral counselling and other options. A client information sheet would therefore be appropriate, including for pre-marital counselling. It should define the types of counselling offered within the church setting (for example, peer, pastoral, and so on); duration of counselling (for example, three sessions only); location; any financial arrangements; counsellor availability; and it should name the credentialing organisation whose ethical code binds the counsellor.

Pastoral best practice and ethics require that notes are taken during or immediately after counselling sessions. Given the public nature of many pastoral counsellors' offices, such records must be kept securely locked or password-protected.

In the end, church-based counselling is not a hard science. In the 6th century, Gregory the Great wrote: "The government of souls is the art of arts" (as cited in Culbertson & Shippee, 1990). But like all artistic endeavours, the structure, including its ethics, which underlies the art, is what guarantees the beauty and satisfaction of the final product.

3.8 MANAGING COMPLEX RELATIONSHIPS IN LESBIAN, GAY, BISEXUAL, TRANSGENDER AND INTERSEX COMMUNITIES

Antony McFelin

This section examines some of the matters that lesbian, gay, bisexual, transgender and intersex (LGBTI) counsellors might consider when they are relating to LGBTI clients. In particular, it focuses on the value of responsible caring (NZAC, 2002). Responsible care in counselling includes maintaining boundaries and working within the limits of one's competence. However, the complex nature of LGBTI communities often makes it difficult to separate personal from professional involvement. There is no question that multiple relationships are a common reality for practitioners working in LGBTI communities:

> ... we believe that practitioners must remain flexible when deciding whether to engage in multiple relationships with a client. We also believe that it is important for practitioners working in LGBT communities to develop their own networks for consultation and support. (Kessler & Waehler, 2005)

The LGBTI community is a diverse group in Aotearoa New Zealand. Despite social changes since homosexual law reform in 1986, there are still instances of prejudice or open hostility towards LGBTI people. This difficult context amplifies the importance of trust and understanding when LGBTI clients seek a counsellor. Not only must a counsellor be able to demonstrate caring intent, a respectful attitude towards LGBTI clients, and a responsible professional approach, but they must also demonstrate their trustworthiness, particularly in "respect[ing] the confidences with which they are entrusted" (4.4). With trust, respect and competence in mind, LGBTI clients may prefer to work with LGBTI counsellors. Others may seek counselling from outside the LGBTI community. Responsible caring interweaves with the value of personal integrity (3.5) and respect for human dignity (3.1).

RELATEDNESS DURING COUNSELLING

The central concern of this discussion is the matter of privacy, and of managing the inevitable multiple-role relationships in LGBTI small communities. It is always the responsibility of counsellors, not clients, to "set and monitor the boundaries between a counselling relationship with a client and any other kind of relationship with that client and for making such boundaries as clear as possible for the client" (5.11.c). The discussion that follows both draws on the general points that have been made earlier in this book (Part 3, Section 6) on multiple relationships, and focuses on particular considerations relevant to LGBTI counsellors. For LGBTI counsellors the personal–professional interface offers particular challenges concerning community membership, informed consent, disclosure and personal surprises. Each of these is discussed in turn.

1. INVOLVEMENT IN THE LGBTI COMMUNITY

LGBTI counsellors choose different positions within LGBTI communities, and these can be read differently by potential clients. For example, Syme (2003) stated quite strongly that an LGBTI counsellor is "in danger of being seen as standoffish, of losing credibility and possibly denying their own membership of the ... group" (p. 100) if they are not active within LGBTI communities. On the other hand, questions about the ability to hold confidences and trust may arise when a counsellor is central in a community. Whether a counsellor chooses to facilitate a social gathering or to restrict their socialising to a small group, there will be a constant weighing up of competing imperatives, both for themselves and their clients.

The following are relevant questions for LGBTI counsellors to consider.

1. *What roles will I have with LGBTI clients?* LGBTI counsellors may develop roles as counsellor, support person, support group facilitator, and, perhaps also, social network provider. It is important to consider which roles are therapeutically important, how these roles will interact, and how they might impinge on

personal lives. At the outset of counselling, it is important to talk through the differences between social support and the counselling role.

2. *If I am involved in the community, and engage in mutual support with other LGBTI people in social gatherings, what are my responsibilities when a client joins the same social networks?*

3. *If there is an open invitation to a gathering at a LGBTI counsellor's home, because social support is seen as important, what will I do if a client arrives?* If an LGBTI counsellor is in the practice of providing social network opportunities for the LGBTI community, the effects of offering their own home as a gathering place for social support and networking should be considered.

4. *If I am working with a client who is on the journey of coming out, will I have any role beyond the counselling room?* For example, it is important to discern whether to link a client who is experiencing isolation to support networks of which I may myself be a member (Kessler & Waehler, 2005). If I do not actively offer this support, what happens when a client, on the invitation of someone else, joins a social group to which I belong?

5. *If I have a partner, what discussions might be important in anticipating the kinds of situations outlined above, so as not to compromise my professional responsibilities?* How will I manage the complex interaction of social relationships while protecting professional and personal relationships? For example, how might I think about the possibility that, at social gatherings, my partner might unknowingly meet a client of mine and suggest to this person we might all meet up again in a social context?

Many LGBTI counsellors prefer caution, and do not enter compromising situations that may lead to confusing or ambiguous messages about the part they might play in a client's personal life. A test for what is appropriate participation and involvement in the community may be the reactions of professionals around us. With a supervisor or other trusted counselling colleagues, we can explore and evaluate whether our involvement in social support is compromising responsible care in the counselling relationship. It may also be appropriate to check out with clients how they are affected. A robust understanding and experience in managing these roles and responsibilities provides a solid foundation for talking with clients about potentially overlapping relationships. The next section looks at this practice in further detail.

2. INFORMED CONSENT

Whatever roles LGBTI counsellors take, it is important to prepare themselves and LGBTI clients for potential dual/multiple roles, as part of the process of informed consent. For example, an LGBTI counsellor might suggest, as their preferred practice, that whenever there are gatherings where they are likely to meet, or in the situation of an unexpected meeting, the counsellor will not initiate contact. Based on the principle of responsible caring, an LGBTI counsellor may need to be very explicit about the types of unexpected encounters that may occur. It may also be important to tell clients that others in the community might ask about how a counsellor and client know each other. From first contact, and as therapeutic relationships develop, the uneven distribution of power implicit in the counselling relationship places the responsibility on counsellors to make visible possible pitfalls that may not be visible to clients. It is important to reiterate that counsellors will always carry a professional responsibility for monitoring and maintaining boundaries between professional and other relationships.

3. DISCLOSURE

Thus far the assumption has been that both counsellor and client know from the outset of therapeutic contact that each identifies as LGBTI. However, this might not be the case. Disclosure raises significant questions relevant to the safety of clients or counsellors.

1. *Do I routinely disclose my preferred sexual identity, as part of the way I present myself as a professional counsellor, to all clients?* What are the benefits for counsellor and clients of such disclosure? What are the risks? As in every counselling situation, counsellor disclosure should not override an LGBTI client's experiences or concerns.

2. *If I do not routinely disclose, how will I respond if a client then tells me during counselling that they are LGBTI; or that they are struggling against taking up an LGBTI identity; or are pained because someone they care about has recently come out or taken up LBGTI identity?* Will I then disclose my own sexual identity? If so, when might it

be appropriate to do so and why? What effects might there be for the therapeutic relationship?

3. *If I do not disclose, and later meet a client at an LGBTI social event where my sexual identity is clear, what impact will this have on our counselling relationship?*

4. *If a client has not told me of their sexual identity, and I meet them in a social situation where their sexual identity is clear, what response should I make, either in the moment, or at the next counselling session?*

5. *If I do not routinely disclose, how will I respond if a client expresses some antipathy towards LGBTI people?* When the intensity of negative attitude is high, a carefully considered decision is needed. Because such moments can have great significance for counselling relationships, it is important for counsellors to weigh up very carefully, in advance, the competing responsibilities of care and social justice. Any response needs to ensure that the engagement in the relationship continues if possible.

4. OVERLAPPING RELATIONSHIPS AND INTIMACY

Because LGBTI communities are small, often supportive and close, overlapping relationships are difficult to avoid. The complexities of different levels of intimacy, relevant to any counselling community, are heightened. In particular, situations might arise involving clients and the sexual exposure of LGBTI counsellors that could threaten or damage the work of counselling. These situations are difficult to resolve and point to the importance of good supervision.

1. Gabriel and Davies (2000) explored a challenging situation with uncompromising clarity. They asked what happens when an anonymous sexual encounter occurs and the LGBTI counsellor realises that the other person is a client? They suggested that the LGBTI counsellor, in the moment, ends the encounter and seeks permission to explore, at the next counselling session, what has happened. This response enacts the NZAC *Code of Ethics* call to "assume full responsibility for setting and monitoring the boundaries" (5.11.a). However, since the counsellor is also prohibited from sexual relationships with current clients (5.13.a), there is a further responsibility. The counsellor should disclose

this encounter to their supervisor and consider responsibility for reporting the incident to the Ethics Secretary.

Gabriel (2005) suggested a three-stage process to be used in such unexpected situations. The first stage is to deal with the shock of the situation and contain it through dialogue with the client. The next stage involves discussing and processing the situation with the client at the next counselling session if any such counselling session should take place. In the third stage the LGBTI counsellor should process the issues in supervision and/or personal counselling.

2. What happens when an LGBTI counsellor meets a client's partner, and realises that they have been in a romantic and/or sexual relationship with the partner? How is the counselling relationship affected, especially if there are difficult feelings between the now-former partner and the LGBTI counsellor?

3. What if a client comes to a counsellor with whom they have had a previous sexual relationship? The client wants to see someone of the same gender and, in that particular counselling service, there is no alternative counsellor. The NZAC *Code of Ethics* says: "Counsellors shall not provide counselling to persons with whom they have had a sexual or romantic relationship" (5.13 d). How does a counsellor support this person, especially if the situation is an emergency? It is important that a counsellor is able to offer some support to help the person engage with an appropriate counsellor. In preparation for such a situation, it is advisable to develop a referral network – as indeed it is for all counsellors.

TAKING UP OTHER FORMS OF RELATEDNESS AFTER COUNSELLING

"Counsellors shall not exploit the potential for intimacy made possible in the counselling relationship, even after counselling has ended" (5.13 b): the power relationship is likely to continue between counsellors and those who have been clients, should there be ongoing contact.

1. After the counselling relationship has ended, does the NZAC *Code of Ethics* leave the possibility open for an LGBTI counsellor to form a romantic and/or sexual relationship with their former LGBTI client? If an LGBTI counsellor journeyed through a client's coming out process, would it be possible to later develop

a romantic and/or sexual relationship? The *Code of Ethics* does not explicitly prohibit such relationships, but it is firm in guarding against exploitation. This is the measure. In such situations the counsellor will have learnt much about their client, and counselling is explicitly non-reciprocal in its prioritising of clients' interests.

2. Does the nature of the concern the client took to counselling influence the relationships of power after counselling has ended, and therefore have a less prohibitive effect on the taking up of post-counselling relationships? Would a senior executive, who briefly consults a counsellor about an employment-related opportunity, be considered well-positioned to make an informed decision about a later ongoing social or romantic relationship? What would a counsellor need to consider before proceeding or not?
3. After the counselling relationship is over, is it appropriate for an LGBTI counsellor to suggest that the relationship move to a friendship because of the small and limited situations that clients may have for social support?

Good use of supervision, appropriately open and honest communication with clients, and foresight in planning for possible difficult scenarios are particularly critical for an LGBTI counsellor in maintaining ethical practice. These actions will help counsellors in making balanced decisions, fully aware of the potential for harm that can be caused when power in counselling relationships is misused. A wise counsellor, almost without exception, leaves any initiation of a post-counselling relationship to the client. At the same time, client initiation is no defence for a counsellor who takes up an inappropriate relationship. Because of the power relationship, clients may find it hard to turn down a counsellor's invitation, thus, counsellors who initiate post-counselling romantic or sexual relationships are vulnerable to complaints of sexual harassment (5.13.c). If a counsellor finds that they have thoughts or feelings that might make them consider an invitation to friendship, romance or a sexual relationship with a former client, then they should first turn to their supervisor to explore and understand this, and make a contextually appropriate decision.

3.9 WORKING WITHIN THE SCOPE OF OUR COMPETENCE

Eric Medcalf

Competence involves more than formal qualifications. Welfel (2010) identified three spheres of competence.

1. *Knowledge*: "... being schooled in the history, theory, and research of one's field and cognizant of the limits of current understanding."
2. *Skill*: "... successfully applying interventions with actual clients."
3. *Diligence*: "... a constant attentiveness to the client's needs that takes priority over other concerns" (pp. 81–5).

The NZAC *Code of Ethics* (2002) states that counsellors shall "practice within the scope of their competence" (4.8). It goes on:

> Counsellors shall determine, in consultation with the client, whether they are appropriate to provide the counselling. Where necessary and feasible, counsellors shall refer their clients to other counsellors who would be more appropriate by reason of their skills, gender or culture or for any other reason indicated by the client's needs. (5.3)

And also:

> Counsellors shall work within the limits of their knowledge, training and experience. (5.9.c)

This section addresses some of the issues raised by these statements, and offers some guidance for situations where counsellors may face uncertainty.

WORKING WITHIN KNOWLEDGE LIMITATIONS: CLAIMS TO PARTICULAR COMPETENCIES

In New Zealand counsellors have access to a wide range of professional training and education, from Certificate level to Masters degrees and beyond. They may also undertake training in specific modes and methods of practice. Training may vary from a short one-day seminar to a much longer programme of professional education within the structures provided by an academic or professional institution. The latter may provide graded levels of professional education and training which are assessed and lead to accreditation by the institute. At what point, then, has a counsellor sufficient expertise, in counselling in general or in the use of any particular approach, to claim competence?

Of course counsellors can advertise the types of training they have engaged in, and any levels of accreditation that particular professional education systems may confer. These claims may not always mean much to a client. It is, therefore, a counsellor's responsibility to talk honestly with a client about what their qualifications mean and what the client may expect, especially if the client enquires specifically about a counsellor's competence or professional background. Counsellors should provide documentation – for example a professional disclosure statement (see Judi Miller, Part 2, Section 2) – that offers the client more detail than might be available on a business card or advertisement.

At times prospective clients might approach the counsellor and ask very specific questions, such as, "Do you do CBT?" This inquiry may be fuelled by a referrer's awareness of some research that indicates some effectiveness in the cognitive behavioural treatment of depression, for example. The counsellor may have had a few sessions of learning this modality in their basic qualification or they may have undertaken a lengthy university course devoted entirely to CBT. They may have developed expertise in this approach through independent reading, and supervision from someone who also has expertise. An open conversation about the client's expectations and the counsellor's competence to offer CBT is important here. It may be that the client decides that they can work with the counsellor in respect of their concerns or difficulties, in which case an agreement may be made in full knowledge of the counsellor's competence, or not, in CBT. Alternatively, in the situation where the client counsellor has minimal knowledge the client may be clear that they want a CBT-trained practitioner. In this case the counsellor should help the client find a counsellor who would meet their stated needs.

Before using specific methods, a counsellor should make an adequate assessment that these methods are appropriate. Some techniques may be harmful in certain situations, and counsellors should ensure that they have the competence to make appropriate assessments, when considering the use of such techniques or practices. An example of potential for harm would be the use of relaxation or regressive techniques with clients who are at risk of psychotic regression.

There may be both ethical and legal implications in claiming competence in particular models. For example, increasingly there are trademarked brands of therapy. By way of fictional example, Finckelberg's pro-relate counselling (FPC) methods may require the completion of an extensive and expensive process of accreditation. The use of the name FPC may be proscribed until full accreditation has been achieved. Hence serious legal consequences, as well as questions about honesty and ethics, could arise should a counsellor claim to use these methods after only a brief introductory course.

WHO ARE OUR CLIENTS?

Although a counsellor may have had professional preparation for work with a wide variety of clients, it is likely that their experience, preferences and skill levels will influence, and at times limit, the range of clients they will normally see. Counselling some client groups – children, learning disabled clients and those with severe mental illness, for example – requires particular skills and relevant knowledge, training and supervision. It can also be argued that other areas of practice, such as working with adolescents, people with addiction-related issues, groups, families and couples, also require particular knowledge, skills and experience. What is critical is an evaluation by a counsellor of whether they are competent to offer their services, or whether they should consider referral to another professional with appropriate knowledge and skills or inviting. It may also be appropriate to invite such a person into collaborative practice. Referral, collaborative practice, or consultation may also be necessary where a counsellor's knowledge of the client's culture is not sufficient for the counsellor to offer adequate service.

THE PRACTICE CONTEXT

Counsellors may feel constrained by issues of geographic isolation, or expectations of their role in a work setting. A practitioner might be the only counsellor within a rural community, or a counsellor in a school where they are expected to provide a service to all the students. Here a counsellor, in trying to put into practice the core value of "Responsible Caring" (3.4), is faced with the issue of nothing being available for the client if they do not offer something. Drawing on Hargrove (1986) and Schank and Skovholt (2006), Welfel (2010) stated: "The ethical challenge for rural counsellors and psychotherapists is to provide competent service across a wide range of issues, age groups and populations whilst acknowledging that they are not omnipotent" (p. 93). This is a real issue in New Zealand, where rural counsellors must often be generalists rather than specialists in particular issues. Welfel helpfully brings out the principle of "nonmaleficience," or in the terms of the NZAC *Code of Ethics* "Avoid[ing] doing harm" (4.2) when considering practising at the boundaries of competence. Such work requires that the counsellor be both well supported through supervision and collegiality, and willing and able to extend their competence through professional learning.

In schools it is important that counsellors create and maintain good links with other professionals in both the state and private sectors, who are able to provide the specialist services that often overstretched school counsellors cannot. This point draws into focus the issue of capability versus capacity. A counsellor may be competent to undertake various therapeutic roles with their clients, but organisational constraints might mean that there is not time available, or that other tasks take priority. Good links with external agencies will enable the counsellor to care responsibly by sharing some of their therapeutic challenges with others in the wider community.

THE COUNSELLOR AS AN ADULT LEARNER

Counselling is a process in which both counsellor and client must often face the unknown. It is not an activity where one person *does* something to another to *make them better*. It is a dynamic process where risks may be taken in order to promote and enable positive change. The hope and intention is that both will learn through the encounter – the client becoming more able to face the challenges in their life, and the counsellor becoming more experienced, with increased knowledge, wisdom and skill. So how can we decide on our suitability to work with a client, and in ways that meet our ethical obligation to work within our knowledge limitations?

Kolb's (1984) well-known cycle of adult learning suggests a process of:

concrete experience;
reflective observation;
abstract conceptualisation;
active experimentation.

This is more than just a process of trial and error, and will require access to knowledgeable and challenging support processes, such as a good supervisor. With this opportunity for responsible reflection and possible guidance, a counsellor embarking into unknown territory will be able to extend their competence and the client achieve some benefit. The role of the supervision process is critical here, as a supervisor must work with a counsellor to ensure that the risks are low, and that a counsellor is working within their learning range. In these situations a supervisor has an increased responsibility to help a counsellor to manage the ethical boundaries of their work: the risks must be scaffolded within ethical frameworks.

The ethical guideline of informed consent (5.5) also has clear relevance here. If a counsellor is working at the boundaries of their competence then they will consider the possibility that the client could be involved in making choices about their involvement in such practices. Here a process of ethical decision-making can guide action in terms of the appropriateness of informing the client.

WHEN THE COUNSELLOR'S COMPETENCE IS TEMPORARILY IMPAIRED

Counsellors are human beings and subject to the same rigours of life as anyone else. Amongst other things, we may suffer relationship breakdown, bereavement, accidents and illness. As well, we work with people experiencing stress and vulnerability, which may stretch our emotional resources. We may suffer "vicarious traumatisation" (Pearlman & Saakvitne, 1995). We may burn out (Everall & Paulson, 2004), or suffer impairment or distraction from events in our lives. At times, then, our ability to respond in a skilful, empathic way, and to be diligent, may be impaired. The ethical requirement that we be fit to practice (5.10) links with the ethical responsibility to work within our competence. It is thus important that we, and our colleagues, take into account our limitations, and draw boundaries around our workloads to ensure that we maintain effective services to clients.

The principle of informed consent is worth bearing in mind when a counsellor's practice is impaired because of an event in their own life.

It would rarely be appropriate for a counsellor to share their personal concerns with their client; there is a risk that the client may feel that they have to care for the counsellor. However, denial of the impairment may create a tension in which the client becomes aware that all is not okay with the counsellor but the counsellor responds with: "We're here to talk about you, not me." Some disclosure may help, even if it's just to identify the impairment as arising from personal issues. There may be ethical justification for disclosing issues that have *commonality*, such as the illness of a close relative, as opposed to issues for which a counsellor may feel some personal and professional sensitivity, such as marital or parenting problems. Such dilemmas require thorough consideration, perhaps in supervision, of whether the disclosure has potential for benefit, or harm, and for whom. There are potential dangers when the disclosure is made spontaneously, in the heat of the moment, when the heat is generated from the counsellor's own reaction to the client's story – for example, if a client's disclosure of abuse triggers the counsellor's own experience. On the other hand, the compassionate witnessing (Weingarten, 2003) of a client's story, and appropriate disclosure, can have therapeutic effects when the focus clearly remains on the client's needs.

A temporary withdrawal from work may, in itself, respond to ethical requirements of fitness to practice, and model good self-care. The appropriate provision of counselling by another counsellor is, in that situation, competent practice. Counsellors in group practices may be able to engage a colleague to work with their clients for the duration of their impairment. Others may ask colleagues to provide locum coverage.

As Fran Parkin and Kathie Crocket note (Part 2, Section 3), there is a challenge for self-employed counsellors, when no work means no income. The temptation to work whilst impaired may be great. Income protection insurance may not start until some time after the impairment has begun, and then only if it is something that can be certified by a doctor. It is therefore wise to plan for such a possibility so that counsellors can respond appropriately at a time of impairment.

WHEN THE COUNSELLOR *FEELS* INCOMPETENT

Occasionally when working with a client a counsellor may feel as if they are incompetent. This is different from actually lacking competence. For instance, the client may behave in ways that undermine the counsellor, playing out behaviours which create difficulties in their social relationships generally. The need for adequate collegial support and supervision here is great: a normally skilled and competent counsellor may experience themselves as deskilled in a client's attempts to hold onto a dysfunctional life position. Such collegial support will both affirm the counsellor and offer opportunities to reflect on, understand, and respond, in a highly complex situation.

SUMMARY

Meeting the requirement to work within the limits of competence presents a challenge to counsellors to be open and honest about their experience and the type and length of their training; to be self-aware, honest and realistic; to avoid harmful compromises in the interests of income or status; and to use collegial and supervisory support to the full. It also presents the necessity for a counsellor to adhere to the NZAC *Code of Ethics* 5.9, continuing their education, extending their skills and knowledge, and rethinking what they already know in the light of both their own experience and new developments in research and theory.

3.10 UNBEARABLE AFFECT IN ETHICAL PROBLEMS

Bill Grant

As counsellors we may have the credentials, know the *Code of Ethics*, be highly skilled, and have years of experience, yet we may nevertheless find ourselves in extremely difficult and challenging situations with clients or colleagues. These situations often arise, and persist, as a consequence of difficulties around unbearable affect. The purpose of this section is to suggest some of the ways in which difficulties may arise around unbearable affect and to indicate contexts for dealing with such difficulties to prevent them from growing into complaints, or even court cases.

Affect is rather neglected in much of the discourse about ethics, which tends to deal more with what we think and do, rather than with what we experience with our emotions and bodies. I have come to the conclusion that when things go wrong in counselling relationships, it is often a consequence of an unbearable affective experience. The unbearable experience comes first, tending to be preverbal. The problematic actions or thoughts follow. On the other hand, if the experience *can* be borne in mind, and thought about, then any actions are less likely to be problematic and they may even promote therapeutic progress. This begs the question: how to bear this heavy load that comes with the work of counselling?

Such unbearable experiences can take many forms: I may experience loathing for my client or I may feel that s/he loathes me; I may feel sexually curious or aroused by my client; I may have an urge to help my client in ways that go way beyond normal professional boundaries; I may feel a secret gratification at my client's apparent love for me; my client may indeed fall in love with me and I may find this disturbing. In some situations, I may notice no emotion, but all sorts of bodily experiences may disturb me in the presence of clients: my skin creeping, my stomach churning, my head hurting, my foot tapping, my heart pounding, my leg itching or my fingers scratching at an itch that doesn't really warrant a scratch. I may experience nothing but deadness with a client: a complete absence of affect. And as well as experiences like this, I may feel shame that I am prone to having such experiences with my clients. Although affect is often masked or hidden, it is as real as a scar on the wrist or shattered knuckles.

These experiences are unbearable for several reasons. They tend to be unpleasant, and they may not fit with the picture I have of myself as a counsellor: a credentialed professional working benevolently for troubled people. Hateful feelings about my clients seem unprofessional, are unthinkable, unbearable. As well, I may not have learned how to contain such powerful experiences. I cannot bear them because I don't know how to. The way I once learned to bear bad experiences was to take them to my parents with whom I may have found some soothing, some words to put to my experience, and some thoughts with which to converse and begin to build an understanding within which to hold my experience. This is perhaps the original confessional and cleansing ritual. But it can be a challenge to both our courage and resourcefulness to find ways of engaging in such processes within our adult professional lives.

Affect is relational. It is experienced by each of us bodily, but it is mediated in the relational field between people. These people may be the people in the room, but there may be other people contributing to my experience. My own mother died thirty years ago, but sometimes, if a new client has a particular way of taking her seat, a particular dark colouring of wavy hair, a certain lilt in her voice, or a way of looking out the window, I can have a feeling that my mother, or maybe some aspect of her, is in the room with us. And with this comes a momentary sense of reverie that comes from some time in my early childhood. This is no problem; I recognise the trigger and quickly establish the unique qualities of my client, while my fragment of Mum takes her place quietly behind me. She can still chip in occasionally. But such triggers can be distressing as well as enhancing.

One of the first to write about the complexity of affect in the counselling room was Ferenczi (1955), who wrote of his discovery of the way many clients struggled with negative feelings about him, as well as of his own varied feelings about his clients. He found that by incorporating this new knowledge into his practice with care, he enabled his work with such clients to become unstuck. Ferenczi's discovery brought some hitherto unbearable and unspeakable experiences into the light of the known world in the counselling room. More than this, he welcomed them as resources, as active participants in the client's healing.

In the same paper, Ferenczi brought another important discovery out of the darkness: that real sexual trauma in childhood, as distinct from memories of childhood fantasies, plays an important role in the development of mental health problems. One could say that the actions of client and counsellor in bringing a story of abuse out of the darkness and into the space between them is the beginning of healing. Maybe it is also the beginning of ethics. It requires courage. The myth of Tane is about this process of going into a dark place despite fear, and bringing back knowledge, so expanding *te ao marama*, the world of light, the known world (O'Connor & Macfarlane, 2002; Reed, 2004). Accident Compensation counsellors working with clients who were sexually abused as children experience the central part played by affect in this work.

It is difficult to write and think about affect in the same kind of way as it is difficult to write and think about tastes and scents. Like wine in the mouth, affect is experienced rather than thought. Thinking *about* affect is not the same as experiencing it, although thinking plays an essential part in the management of difficulties with affect. We have to translate an experience into the symbolic material that is the stuff of thought.

According to a psychodynamic perspective, the foundations of this symbolic representation of affect appear to be laid in the noisy, redolent wrestling of parent and baby. Peek-a-boo is one of the first dramas and it contains the elements of affect regulation that may see us through the other dramas of life. In peek-a-boo we can learn that those powerful feelings that erupt within us are real, that they are shared by someone who has a grasp of what we are experiencing, that they can be given names (including "baby names"), so we may start to think about them, and know that they can be managed, or even played with.

Peek-a-boo has similarities with good, ethical counselling. The drama of counselling practice, however, makes one vulnerable to occasionally losing the ability to name what we may be feeling, to think and talk about affect, to bear it in mind. For example, a client enters and I am instantly aware of his overwhelming affective presence. I may not know what it is, but I experience it, together with some of my reactive fear. My first impulse is to unload the unbearable burden he has suddenly put on me. I create a barrier between my experience and my awareness. I dissociate.

So I may smile, or press on with operational business, or do other things to cover what is going on affectively between us. Most clients are able to cope with being related to in this way, perhaps because it is a behavioural style which they have come to expect from professional people. A tacit agreement is made between us, to dissociate jointly from this affective relationship so that we can press on with business. Work gets done, sure enough, but it is done without the involvement of the disaffected parts of us, which hover like two ghosts in the corners. My client, of course, notices that a vital, if unnamed, part of him is beyond my comfort zone, and this can serve to exclude that aspect of his life from the therapeutic process, thereby limiting its potential effectiveness for the client.

When a counsellor acts out unethically the local counselling community can have trouble dealing with affect, which can compound the damage. Private doubts about a colleague's practice or fitness to practice often go unexpressed. Unease, ambivalence, fear, shame and other strong emotional reactions can inhibit us from engaging in frank discussion with one another. Without talking, thinking is disabled, and nothing gets done to protect clients, the counsellor, or the profession. I have known a number of counsellors who have been publicly disgraced, professionally censured, or even jailed after ethical breaches. In most cases, some colleagues had harboured private concerns about certain aspects of these counsellors' work, but nothing effective was done to translate the inner concern into professional thought and discussion, and so facilitate engagement with, and containment of, the issues.

Even when difficulties do reach the light of day, there remain a number of challenges for how a counselling community manages affective responses. After each drama has passed its climax, there still needs to be a proper dénouement. If the protagonist has gone, there remain some stunned and saddened colleagues who need to acknowledge the truth and damage, to bear it in mind. My hope is that as NZAC and other professional bodies develop more effective complaints processes, earlier recognition and containment of problems at a local level will lead to better repair and prevention.

All of this means that we as counsellors have a particular need to be able to bear affect. In addition, we need to find ways of naming, thinking and talking about the unspoken affective transactions that take place constantly between people. The most important way of attending to these needs in professional life is by having regular supervision with a supervisor who is well attuned affectively; who goes beyond the cognitive and incorporates attending to feelings as part of attending to the whole person of the counsellor within the process of supervision, and who is willing and able to bring up the unbearable questions. Practitioners who have been convicted after legal as well as ethical breaches often reveal that they had not talked about problematic affective issues in their supervision. Alternatively, when supervisors enable us as counsellors to engage in supervision with all dimensions of our experiences with clients, including the affective, we are together promoting mindful and ethical counselling. Through this process we, in turn, are enabled to bring new understandings into the counselling space in a way that promotes the health of the client.

Counsellor education has a significant role to play in equipping counsellors to deal with the challenging affective experiences inherent in the work. Trainees need to develop a high level of awareness of their own feelings and affective experiencing, as well as the capacity to discern and respond effectively to others' affect, and they need to be equipped to use the language of affect in relation to themselves, their clients, and their group. There is a danger that counselling training may privilege cognition and behaviour. Affect should be one of the leading players, rather than a bit-part serving the stars, if graduates are to be adequately prepared to work effectively with clients.

Training and professional development for working with affect can take many forms. A significant experience of personal counselling can enhance trainees' awareness of their own feelings, and their capacity to acknowledge and manage their affective styles, responses, and personal processing within their professional work. For many years in Dunedin I enjoyed being a member of a very diverse counsellors' reading group. We did our reading aloud, there and then in the group, taking turns, and regularly interrupting the flow of the text to question, tell an anecdote, quibble, free associate, and so on. I valued the contribution of this group as a professional community in which I could hone my relationship with affect.

In our practice as counsellors, ethical issues arise from relationships in which affect plays a central part. Thinking about unbearable affect is hard work because it involves thinking about the unthinkable. Some people can manage life without doing this very much, but a counsellor can't.

3.11
PHYSICAL TOUCH IN COUNSELLING RELATIONSHIPS

Irene Esler and Carol White

TO TOUCH OR NOT TO TOUCH?

In counselling relationships, touch is a complex matter. Shaking hands, for example, may be a common social custom, but when is offering to shake a client's hand appropriate or not? Touch is imbued with cultural meanings. When the possibility of physical contact occurs within counselling relationships, counsellors should consider both their intentions and the potential effects of their actions. The meanings clients make of the experience of touch within a therapeutic relationship determines whether the effect of touch may be therapeutic or unhelpful and potentially damaging. Touch is therefore an area of practice that requires careful and ongoing ethical consideration.

BOUNDARIES AND THE POWER RELATION IN COUNSELLING

A counsellor is responsible for establishing and maintaining safe physical and psychological boundaries because of the relations of power inherent in the professional counselling relationship (NZAC, 2002, 5.1.a & b; 5.11.a). Take the examples of a client finding it difficult to refuse a hug initiated by a counsellor, or a client requesting inappropriate touch. In both instances – and always – the responsibility lies with the counsellor to consider the effect of such touch on the client and to manage the situation. Because of the potential effects, and because of the possibility of such touch being misunderstood by clients, counsellors are advised to err on the side of caution. As McNeil-Haber (2004) stated, "Ethical consideration of the use of appropriate touch lies in the ethical principle that above all therapists should do no harm and avoid exploitation" (p. 137).

WHAT KINDS OF TOUCH MIGHT BE ACCEPTABLE?

Questions about appropriate touch cannot be answered without reference to the cultural context. Erotic touch is clearly inappropriate in the context of professional counselling relationships in any cultural context. In this section, we focus on the kinds of physical contact that, in Western cultures, might be commonly thought of as non-sexual, such as a hand-shake, a touch on the arm, shoulder or back, or a hug.

There is a range of opinion in the professional literature regarding touch within counselling relationships. Some authors advocate the avoidance of touching as much as possible: "Many would warn against the use of touch in a professional setting because touch for many of our clients has been used to hurt or exploit" (Strozier, Krizek & Sale, 2003, p. 49). Nevertheless, Zur and Nordmarken (2006) reported surveys that suggested that most therapists hug their clients or approve of the appropriate use of touch, while Tune's (2001) study noted that touch in the "social space" at the beginning or end of a counselling session was less likely to be questioned by therapists than touch in the "therapeutic space" of the session itself (p. 169). However, as Tune (2008) later noted, such a distinction ignores the continuity of therapeutic relationship and responsibility.

Two decades ago, Willison and Masson's (1986) review of the research and clinical literature on the value of therapeutic touch suggested that "touch facilitates the counselling process by increasing the client's positive evaluation of the experience" (p. 499). Their position was moderated by the addition of cautions, and detail of times when touch should not be used. These cautions align with the guidelines offered below. Later, Hunter and Struve (1998) argued that touch is a fundamental need, and as such is intrinsic to the therapeutic process, while Hetherington (1998) suggested that refraining from the appropriate use of touch in the counselling situation also has the potential for harm. Welfel (2006) reported that there is no clear research evidence to clarify the situation with respect to non-erotic touch in counselling. Responsible practice depends, therefore, on counsellors' ongoing ethical decision-making in order to take ongoing judicious actions in professional practice settings.

TOUCH AND CULTURAL MEANINGS

Physical contact in the counselling relationship comes layered with many meanings, depending on one's culture, socialisation and individual experience (Zur & Nordmarken, 2006). For example, Māori clients may expect to greet with a kiss, handshake, or a hongi, while Muslim women and men will likely refrain from shaking hands with a person of a different gender.

PROFESSIONAL EDUCATION AND THE ETHICS OF TOUCH

A study of social workers in the United States (Strozier et al., 2003), suggested that they had received little education, training or supervision in the use of touch. Willison and Masson (1986) noted that the emphasis in counsellor training is on verbal communication. Could it be that this is also the experience for most of us? How much did the ethics of touch in the counselling relationship feature in your own counsellor education? A lack of specific training could account for another commonly held response: that therapists rely on their intuition, justifying touch on the basis that "I touch if it 'feels right.'" We advise that this kind of justification is not sufficient. In any situation where counsellors touch clients, we should be able to give a clear account of our purposes. We offer some guidelines below to support your consideration of how you use touch in your counselling practice. These are intended as general guidelines, and do not specifically address any approach to counselling that employs touch as a specific therapeutic technique.

COMPLAINTS IN NEW ZEALAND: WHAT CAN WE LEARN?

Inappropriate touching or misunderstandings around touching have formed the basis for some complaints against NZAC counsellors. Of the 104 complaints made to NZAC between 1991 and 2000, six were specifically about inappropriate touch, and ten were about sex with the client (Winslade & White, 2002). While these data refer to complaints not findings, the point to be taken is that touch has been a recurrent cause for concern amongst clients. Touch is an area of practice that requires careful and ongoing ethical consideration.

SOME SUGGESTED GUIDELINES

The following guidelines for considering the ethics of touch in counselling relationships draw on Hunter and Struve (1998):

- The purpose of the touch appears to be as clear as possible to both people;
- Touch is intended to benefit the client and to serve his or her interests, and the counsellor has considered possible effects. It is therefore not based on persuasion or domination;
- The counsellor has checked that the client wants to be touched, and the client is in a position to decline (see, for example, Kitzinger, 2000);
- The therapeutic relationship has developed sufficiently so that meanings around the intention and the effects of touch can be discussed;
- The counsellor could view a video of what transpired and account for the touch as demonstrating respect for human dignity, and responsible caring;
- The counsellor is able to differentiate between clients in their use of touch, and can satisfactorily account for the appropriateness of the differentiation;
- The counsellor is comfortable with touch.

SOME USEFUL QUESTIONS

These are some further questions that come out of our reading of the literature on touch, and from our own practice as counsellors:

- What kind of touch is acceptable, and in what circumstances?
- What is the cultural context, and what are the implications?
- When is it not acceptable to touch a client?
- Under what circumstances would I hug a client if the hug were initiated by the client?
- What would I need to take into account before I made the decision to initiate a hug with a client? For example, how are these situations different: a client initiating a hug, or a counsellor initiating a hug?
- Whose needs are being met by the touching?
- Is this client special to me? If so, in what way? What difference might this make?

- Is the meaning I associate with this experience of touch the same as the meaning it has for my client, and how would I know?

WHAT DIFFERENCE WOULD IT MAKE IF ...?

In thinking about the ethics of our practice, we find that it is often helpful to ask "What difference would it make if ...?" This question takes us out of the particulars of a situation to help us see what might be visible when taking a broader view. Thinking about touch, what difference would it make if:

- the client and counsellor differ from one another in gender or sexual orientation – and does this question assume that same sex touching does not require the same scrutiny?
- the client and counsellor are different in other ways: culture, age, size, social status, for example?
- the touch is initiated by the client?
- the client requests more touch than the counsellor feels comfortable giving?
- the touch is initiated by the counsellor?
- the touch occurs in the privacy of the counsellor's office or outside the counsellor's office?

THINKING IN PRACTICE: A CONVERSATION ABOUT TOUCH

It is feasible that any of us could find ourselves in a situation where we felt uncomfortable with the degree or extent of the touching within a particular counselling relationship. We believe that noticing even a small discomfort or question is a critical step. The next critical step is how we respond to what we notice.

Tune's (2001) exploratory study suggested that counsellors are more likely to talk about touch in supervision when the touch is client-initiated. We suggest that counsellor-initiated touch is also important for consideration in supervision. In the following scenario, a female counsellor working with a female client notices that hugging is becoming more and more prolonged at the conclusion of each session. The counsellor decides to bring to supervision her questions about what she has noticed.

Supervisor: When did you decide that hugging this client was okay?

Counsellor: At the end of our first session when she asked me for a hug. I never gave it much thought. I'm a huggy kind of person.

Supervisor: What was that decision based on?

Counsellor: When I was in therapy my counsellor hugged me, and it was a non-verbal way of connecting, which I liked, so I assumed that my client would like it too.

Supervisor: How was the decision to hug negotiated with your client?

Counsellor: Well, actually, I didn't discuss it with the client; I didn't give it much thought at all. I realise as I am talking about it now that it is a common practice that I have.

Supervisor: You say it's a common practice. I wonder, what does it mean for your client that you are hugging her?

Counsellor: I don't know what it means for her ... But I realise now that I do want to know, as I think it's got confused.

Supervisor: It's got confused? What does the hugging mean for you?

Counsellor: Well, the meaning seems to have changed for me. I feel uncomfortable now – especially since the last session when the hug was so prolonged, I felt really uncomfortable and uneasy.

Supervisor: Can you say more about those feelings of discomfort and unease?

Counsellor: I feel the client might get the wrong idea. That the hugs may mean something different for her, that the relationship will become muddy with over-friendliness or even sexual attraction. I don't want to encourage that direction in any way.

Supervisor: And what do you think the likelihood might be of these feelings of discomfort affecting the counselling relationship?

Counsellor: Well, now that we are talking about it, I realise that my discomfort could affect the counselling relationship. I could end up thinking about the hugging all through the next session, wondering if she is going to ask me for another hug, and so being more distant because of it.

Supervisor: Do you have any sense of what might be involved in the management of your feelings so that they don't overshadow the work of counselling?

Counsellor: I didn't, but now that we're talking, I think that what I've noticed is really useful. When I think about this client, I think I could go and explore and discuss with her what it has meant for her to be hugged by me, for us to hug, at the end of the session. I will want to be clearer through a discussion about the dilemmas that hugging presents.

Supervisor: What would your hopes be if you have such a discussion?

Counsellor: My hopes would be that we work towards a shared understanding and interpretation of what the hugs are contributing to the counselling, if anything, and that this is made transparent, and remains open for further discussion if needed. This is my responsibility, to initiate this discussion and to gently ask these questions. My intention is to enable us to move forward in the best interests of the counselling work. Another hope would be to invite my client to be able to notice, and voice, what is happening for her in regard to touch or hugs between us, without any experience of blame or responsibility.

CONCLUSION

Rather than mandating no touch under any circumstances, we are advocating that counsellors reflect on the meanings and effects of any physical contact for both ourselves and our clients. Such reflection should take into account particular cultural or gendered meanings of touch, and other differences noted above. Some forms of touch may be used as an appropriate social convention, such as shaking hands, or awhi or hongi for Māori or Pasifika clients. Touch may be used to support a client in response to grief, distress, or anguish, if this is assessed as appropriate at the time. At other times, touch may be an expression of genuinely spontaneous, shared delight in developments a client has made in their life.

The literature supports our position that the more intimate the touch the greater the potential for that touch to be harmful. Our hope is that counsellors will be thoughtful around matters of physical touch with clients and will always be prepared to regard touch as an important aspect of practice to consider in supervision.

3.12
WHEN A CLIENT DIES

Rhonda Pritchard

Counsellors are human beings in relationships of responsible caring for clients. The death of a client is likely to be distressing, even if, in the case of a client with a terminal illness, the death is expected. If the death is sudden, or the result of suicide or homicide, the responses are almost inevitably going to be more varied and more complicated. We may be affected by the death in ongoing and possibly quite surprising ways.

Whatever the cause of death there is always good reason for debriefing – perhaps continuing over time – with supervisor, manager and/or colleagues to talk through the emotional responses to the shock and loss, and questions that arise from the death. Personal counselling may also be valuable in helping us cope and adjust, especially if there is a suicide or homicide. The search for understanding becomes a major part of a grieving process if the client committed suicide, and, if the death is from homicide, there may be traumatic effects as well (Rando, 1993).

When a death is from suicide, it is important to distinguish between responsibility and accountability. We are not responsible for the death of a client, but we are accountable as one of probably a number of key people who were engaged with them and had a duty of care. The duty at this stage is to account for ourselves with our supervisor; to reflect honestly and openly on our role in the counselling relationship and our interactions with the client. It is virtually inevitable after a client's suicide that we find ourselves engaging in an internal process of reviewing and questioning everything to do with our relationship with the client: our professional judgements and functioning, as well as our personal and emotional responses and ways of coping. Our belief in our own professional competence can be severely shaken (Agee, 2001). It is especially helpful, therefore, if our colleagues and supervisor can manage to balance both the need for a professional review and the strong need we have for support, while avoiding an understandable impulse to reassure us unconditionally.

Debriefing serves at least two purposes. One is to fulfil our duty of self-care, as a way to observe the principle of "fitness to practice" (NZAC, 2002, 5.10.a; 5.10.b). We also have the duty to honour the principles to "avoid doing harm" and to "promote the safety and well-being of individuals" by reviewing and reflecting on the counselling we provided to the client (4.2; 4.5). We may have some regrets or concerns about how we responded to the client. In the case of a suicide we may struggle to understand why, despite the hope and commitment that seemed apparent in the therapeutic relationship, the client has taken this final step. We may feel responsible, fear others' judgements, and implicitly blame ourselves, despite rationally knowing that this is unrealistic (Agee, 2001). It is important to review the circumstance around the client's death and check the adequacy of the steps we took if the risk was clear. If the risk was not clear, we may need to review the adequacy of the assessment and service we provided. The least we can do is to take the opportunity to see if any learning from this situation might contribute to an improved level of understanding, protection and care for clients in the future.

This debriefing process, which is ethically responsible, can serve to strengthen counselling practice and restore professional self-confidence, as well as fostering a counsellor's personal development, because the personal and professional effects of client suicide are interrelated (Agee, 2001). The need for consultation and debriefing is likely to be both immediate and ongoing. There may be a range of immediate responsibilities to which we must attend, including responding to the cultural context.

For example, in schools and other educational institutions, the death of a student or colleague may suddenly require the counsellor to put everything else aside to attend to individuals and groups who are affected, to a greater or lesser extent, by the tragedy. Remembering the ethical principles, it is helpful to consider how the values of respect for human dignity, partnership, autonomy and responsible caring might be applied, with awareness and acknowledgment of cultural and other differences. At the very least, counselling might be offered, even recommended, but no one should ever be urged to engage in counselling.

A funeral or tangi can be an opportunity for the counsellor to honour, join and mourn with others who were involved with the person. It is important to use judgement about whether to attend, depending on the attitude of those close to a client who has died; and if welcome, what role to play. Generally, a quiet unobtrusive role is recommended. This gives the counsellor a time and a place to be another human being who is also sad, and who cares.

Over time, there could be legal and other ethical issues to address, particularly in the case of suicide or homicide. There may be a request or summons to give evidence at an inquest or to disclose information or notes to the police or the court, or to the family of a deceased client. While the NZAC *Code of Ethics* does not give any specific guidance about confidentiality in respect of a client who has died, the generally agreed presumption is that confidentiality continues beyond death. The value of this presumption is that clients are more likely to feel safe to disclose their private selves if they feel the disclosures will stay permanently private.

But, as with any ethical dilemma, there may be other principles and needs to weigh up and consider. The Coroner, for example, has a duty to determine the cause of death and the legal powers to require answers to questions; a counsellor may be in the unique position to provide the most relevant information. Seeking legal advice is recommended. For example, it may be possible to ask the Coroner to waive their power to require specific answers, or to restrict questioning to matters which are of central importance to the court's focus of concern. Bond (2000), a United Kingdom authority on standards and ethics, suggested that "a counsellor might feel willing to answer questions in general terms about a client being depressed because of relationship difficulties, but may know there are some things which the client had stressed as being confidential, such as specific feelings about a named sexual partner or a relative" (2000, p. 111).

Members of a client's family may have an understandable desire to talk with a counsellor. This may simply be part of their quest for information and understanding. While the confidentiality of the client's story is one principle to honour, a compassionate response might be to share any information that might be appropriately given that could be of comfort to, or contribute to the understanding of the family. If that is not possible, it would be wise simply to show empathy for them, and to explain the importance of the confidentiality of the relationship.

The family member's approach to a counsellor may arise out of grief-stricken anger, and a wish to investigate and challenge. Silence can be interpreted as defensiveness or hostility. In this case it is wise to seek advice from a supervisor and a lawyer. A carefully worded, restrained and respectful letter may be an appropriate way to respond. Grief takes many forms, and when a client dies, counsellors have a responsibility to monitor our own responses, at the same time as we may be called upon to care for families or communities, or, in the case of homicide or suicide, to take part in legal processes.

3.13
COMMUNICATING WITH OTHER PROFESSIONALS: REFERRAL AND OTHER PRACTICES

Bob Manthei

This section discusses the ethics of respectful communication with other professionals, whilst maintaining respectful relationships with the client at the centre of this communication. Both consultation and referral are considered, taking account of the fact that counsellors may refer to one another, or to a member of other helping or health professions, just as these professions may also make referrals to, or consult with, counsellors. Some of the ethical values that guide counsellors in these collaborative communications are partnership, including partnership with clients; respect; responsible caring; and, wherever possible, respecting client autonomy regarding the ultimate decision. Relevant principles are: Treaty principles, acting with care and respect, increasing clients' ranges of choices, honesty and trustworthiness, competence. Relevant aspects of the NZAC *Code of Ethics* are: 5.3; 5.5.e; 5.9.c; 5.14; 6.2.b; 7.4.a (2002).

CONSULTING WITH OTHER PROFESSIONALS

There are times when a situation arises in which a counsellor might consider communicating with other professionals in order to optimise the help we are able to provide for our clients. Reasons for doing this can include:

- wanting to gain a better understanding of the client's situation;
- needing information about a client's previous involvement with other helping professionals, medical treatment, or condition;

- clarifying who else is involved with the client and in what specific ways;
- wanting to coordinate the efforts of several service providers;
- investigating making a referral to another agency or professional, including inquiring about the availability and suitability of a particular service and checking on the procedure for referring a client for additional help.

This last reason is a common occurrence, and a counsellor can have a number of reasons for thinking about referring by:

- recognising that counsellor and client appear to be incompatible and that a fruitful therapeutic relationship is not developing;
- reaching the limits of one's competence and looking for more specialised or otherwise appropriate help;
- wanting to access a service for the client that might be more culturally appropriate;
- recognising that counselling has been demonstrably ineffective;
- responding to a request from a client for another counsellor.

There are a number of ethical considerations relevant to referral. While making a referral is a form of effective practice that involves constructive professional collaboration, it may nevertheless be associated with some sense of personal or professional failure, which can induce reluctance or hesitation. It can be valuable to discuss, in supervision, ambivalence about communicating with other professionals. One should explore decision-making processes, including weighing up the relevant ethical considerations and the best interests of the client.

There are a number of factors that can inhibit, or even prohibit, this communication with other professionals:

- not wanting to admit one's limits;
- seeing referral as failure;
- anxiety that others will have doubts about one's competence;
- a lack of knowledge about the specific services available;
- being unsure about the competence of certain practitioners or service providers;

- previous negative experiences when communicating with other professionals or referring a client;
- professional isolation;
- being overly possessive and protective toward one's clients and one's own reputation;
- not recognising when consulting other professionals is indicated;
- professional bias, rivalry, or misinformation about various service providers;
- 'patch protection'.

In order to be effective in consulting or referring, it is necessary to find out first what services are available locally, and then foster informal contacts with the key people in those areas. Once the benefits of consulting with someone else are confirmed, whether in supervision or through independent decision-making, the next step is to discuss the process with the client. As far as possible, clients should be full participants in all decisions related to their counselling, including the right to agree to such consultation or to refuse it. Thus, in these instances, it is good practice to discuss with clients all relevant information and professional opinions about:

- why consulting with someone else may be necessary;
- what outcome(s) can be expected;
- the potential advantages and disadvantages for the client;
- how contact or referral would be made and when it would be done;
- what specific information about the client would be given to any third party;
- the specific agency/professional(s) involved.

Informing clients about the procedure to be followed will enable them to make an informed decision. After all, they may not want their situation known to others, and in most cases that wish would need to be respected, unless there are concerns for the safety of the client or another person. The NZAC *Code of Ethics* allows exemptions in such circumstances from the requirement to maintain client confidentiality (6.2).

Once the matter has been discussed fully with a client, and permission to proceed is obtained, it is useful to work out a written agreement together that both client and counsellor sign. This simple permission statement sets out what the counsellor can and will do when consulting an outsider. If possible it should be clearly agreed what information is taken outside the counselling relationship and why. The clearer the process, the less likely it will be that actions will be misconstrued or misinterpreted. Also, there will be less chance that the client will feel manipulated or betrayed, and in the case of referral, rejected or abandoned.

REFERRAL

A referral to another service or agency is a specific form of communicating with other professionals, one which is considered and thoughtful. A number of things need to be considered in this process (Manthei, 1997):

1. Check with the agency or professional to ensure that the service(s) they provide is relevant and appropriate to the client's needs.
2. Check that the person providing the service is qualified, experienced and competent.
3. Check that the practitioner or agency is available to see the client and in what time frame.
4. Check on the length of intervention and expected outcomes.
5. Find out the exact procedure that would be followed so the client can be briefed about the arrangements, and any pre-visit anxieties allayed.
6. Do not expect, ask for, nor accept a fee for making the referral.
7. Find out the details of the protocol the agency requires for making a referral – and follow it. Information about the client required or requested by an agency might include a clear statement of needs, a summary of help already given, a request for a specific service or intervention and, importantly, an indication of what the client thinks about the referral.
8. Communicate fully the results of your inquiries to the client and secure his/her permission to proceed.

If a written referral is made, it is usual practice to provide a client with a copy of the referral letter. Some counsellors prefer to write a referral letter with the client (Simblett, 1997).

An additional consideration in this process is to clarify your and the other professional's or agency's ongoing responsibilities to the client after the referral has been made. Depending on the purpose of the referral, it may be that both the referral agency and you, as the referrer, continue working cooperatively and collaboratively. In order to achieve this, it would be important to clarify your respective roles, and which party would retain overall responsibility for the client during and after the referral process.

The following questions may help clarify the processes and responsibilities during and after referral:

1. Whose role is it to provide continuity of contact with, and care for the client, during the referral process, during the service-provision phase and after the service has been completed?

2. While the client is being seen by the outside agency, what are the referral counsellor's specific responsibilities to the client and to the referral agency? Will these responsibilities change over time?

3. How much information – usually in the form of progress reports – will the outside agency provide the referring counsellor, and at what intervals? Has this information-sharing been discussed with the client and an understanding reached?

4. Is there a need for a written agreement, or contract, on these points, or is a verbal agreement sufficiently clear to all?

In summary, when counsellors are communicating with outside professionals and services, clients have the right to be fully informed and their wishes followed. In addition, counsellors and the agencies or professionals with whom they are talking need to be clear about the purpose, the process and their respective roles and responsibilities.

3.14 ONLINE PRACTICES

Jeannie Wright

A prediction: online counselling and supervision will expand in Aotearoa New Zealand as internet connections become faster, cheaper and more widely available. This section focuses on the ethics of practising online, but, for me, the first question seems to be: is it ethical NOT to extend our practice if clients choose computer-mediated communication? Not claiming to be a technical sort of person (Wright, 2007), I suggest that step one in the process of considering working online is to find support from a 'techie' who will ensure firewalls, virus protection and other programmes designed to provide privacy and to support ethical practice in this digital world are up to date.

In this section, I draw on experience in the United Kingdom, offering online counselling using email (Wright, 2007), and research with colleagues using e-practices in a New Zealand student-counselling service (Wright, Gooder & Lang, 2008). I am currently involved in online supervision as both supervisor and practitioner. We use email and sometimes Skype (a free voice-over-internet phone system). As digital platforms develop, such as Google groups and social networking sites, a range of online practices will become better supported by research and professional ethical guidelines. Checking the International Society for Mental Health Online (www.ismho.org) is one way to keep up to date.

Internationally, there are indications of online practice becoming more mainstream. See, for example http://news.bbc.co.uk/2/hi/health/8225567.stm. More 'how to' books have been published (Evans, 2009; Gackenbach, 2007; Jones & Stokes, 2008). The internet crosses national boundaries with ease, of course, but ethical practice requires a careful assessment of the local situation. Let's look at one now (see Aunt Ethica, 2007, p. 25).

> Dear Aunt Ethica
>
> A client ("Lesley") has asked about online counselling and I hope you can help with the ethical implications. I've been working with Lesley face-to-face for several months now but she is moving to Bangkok for a one year contract with her employer. She has been struggling with depression and anxiety since her teenage years and a lot of our therapeutic work has been focussed on enabling her to continue with and succeed in the job, which is very important to her. Lesley has asked if I'll use email to continue our counselling. I am not very technical, but the main problem is I don't know if the NZAC *Code of Ethics* would apply in this situation. How can I continue to work with Lesley whilst she's in another country? I would like to support her, but also want to work as ethically as I can 'at a distance'.
>
> Thank you
>
> Techno-challenged Tim

The situation in Tim's letter raises several ethical questions, which Aunt Ethica answers very thoroughly. Like this chapter, she refers primarily to the NZAC *Code of Ethics* (New Zealand Association of Counsellors, 2002) specifically Section 13 which refers to "counselling and electronic communication," including "email, fax, telephone, voicemail, video conferences, web messages and instant messages."

> Dear Techno-Tim,
>
> Join the club; most of us over a certain age are a bit unsure about how best to make use of our computers! However, it seems inevitable that electronic communication in counselling will increase dramatically. At present the NZAC Code has a small section on this (Section 13), but I suspect we shall need more detailed guidelines before long. In the meantime, you could obtain the new BACP 'Guidelines for online counselling and psychotherapy: Ethical guidelines for practitioners, providers and clients', which you can purchase online from the BACP website http://www.bacp.co.uk/publications/index.html
>
> Does the NZAC Code apply? Yes it does, if you are an NZAC member or applicant. We are bound by the code(s) of the professional association(s) of which we are members, regardless of where we, or our clients, are based.
>
> That said, you need to acknowledge and discuss together before Lesley leaves, the ways in which this stage of your relationship will be different

and how it will be managed. How often will you contact each other? What time delay can be expected between a message and its response? Will you insert comments in her messages or write continuous responses? What will be the back-up arrangements, if you are unable to establish email contact? How do you each expect communication to differ, working at a distance? (There can be advantages as well as disadvantages.) How will payment be calculated and organised? Given the difficulties with anxiety and depression it may be particularly important to discuss how you together will monitor her safety. There is the potential for you to need to help her access additional support (you might need to find someone to consult about mental health systems and attitudes in Bangkok) or to assist in making arrangements for her to get home, if she became really unwell.

Also, discuss with her the issues around ensuring confidentiality. Remember that an ordinary email message is really just an electronic postcard. You can each protect against this by encrypting your messages (sending them in code). Check your existing email application (Outlook, Entourage, Eudora etc) and you may find it already includes an encrypting facility. Alternatively, you can download an encrypting system to link to your email software. If all this sounds too technical, an IT consultant can help. Beyond the mail system however, each of you needs to be aware of potential access to your own computer. Think about family members, work colleagues, curious passers-by in internet cafés or at wireless hotspots in public places. Talk also about whether messages will be stored, and, if so, how. You cannot ensure that your client protects herself, but it is your responsibility to consider the risks with her and that she knows that you have taken care that your computer is secure.

Best wishes for your venture into this form of practice. I think it offers a lot of potential for greater access to counselling.

Aunt Ethica

CHECKLIST FOR ETHICAL PRACTICE

The following checklist about online counselling and supervision using email is based on my practice experience and resources from the International Society for Mental Health Online (www.ishmo.org) including articles free to download, plus the very active New Zealand-based organisation, Netsafe (www.netsafe.org.nz), which has a regular column in the New Zealand Association of Counsellors Newsletter:

- Ensure the computer your client is using is relatively secure. Using internet cafes or workplace computers for online counselling and supervision is not recommended unless encryption is available. Even home computers can be problematic if not password protected.

  This sounds like common sense, and it is like closing the office door for a confidential conversation. How far you can ensure your online clients are taking these fundamental steps towards protecting their online privacy is questionable, however.

- Review and follow legal and ethical counselling codes relevant to the work you are doing.

  Your own professional body, such as NZAC, provides the relevant code, irrespective of where your client is based. Also see www.ismho.org.

- Adapt your usual assessment processes (www.ismho.org) when making initial contact and appointments using online media.

- Inform clients about the use of encryption methods to help ensure confidentiality. As Netsafe has so thoroughly documented, there is no such thing as absolute security online. The limits of confidentiality must be explained to clients.

- Names and details of clients, and other information that means a client could be identified to third parties, should not be used in internet communication.

- 'Deleting' files, emails or even text messages does not mean that those communications have been destroyed.

  Using a data stick may be advisable rather than storing unencrypted communications on your hard drive (see www.netsafe.org.nz).

- Inform clients if sessions are being supervised and if and how session transcripts are being preserved by the counsellor/supervisor.

  This is ethical practice in any setting.

- Resist the temptation to forward client email messages (very easy to do informally or casually) to other referral sources without client consent.

- Inform clients if, how, and for how long electronic session transcripts are being preserved.
- Encourage clients who wish to keep a record of sessions to do so in a confidential manner.
  Your control over these decisions is limited.
- Explain to clients the possibility of technological failure, such as what to do if an email message is lost, a password forgotten or a computer breaks down. Back-up systems, for example using the telephone, need to be negotiated.
  It is always wise to ensure you have clients' contact details, for example their cell phone number, for any eventuality.
- Explain to clients how to deal with potential misunderstandings arising from the lack of visual cues between client and counsellor.
  The 'how to' books (Evans, 2009; Jones & Stokes, 2009) are excellent sources of advice on these issues.
- Provide links to appropriate accreditation agencies.
  Let your clients know about your professional membership and accreditation.

SUMMARY

The shift towards online counselling support and self-help is moving fast. Innovative moves by some New Zealand Government ministries, with the award-winning, self-help site 'thelowdown' aimed at young people (www.thelowdown.org.nz) as an excellent example, are worth studying so that you can pass on to online clients the best of the "stand alone" computerised systems. Sound practice-based guides will support the development of competence in offering online counselling, group work and supervision. There is a wealth of detailed information in the referenced texts, covering a far wider range of online applications than this brief section. The ethical question about reaching those who choose not to use face-to-face services is urgent. Ethical practice in online environments by competent practitioners seems to be one way forward.

Acknowledgement

With thanks to Aunt Ethica in *Counselling Today,* September 2007, 30(1), p. 25.

3.15 ELECTRONIC RECORDING OF COUNSELLING CONVERSATIONS

Kathie Crocket

New technologies have made audio and video recording of counselling more accessible, and have expanded the possible contributions of recordings for both clients and counsellors. Exploring the effects of recording devices in research contexts, including counselling, Speer and Hutchby (2003) suggested that recording devices are not necessarily intrusive but can be used in ways that are facilitative of relationships and tasks. Aveline's (1997) advice was that recordings in therapy be "routine and unobtrusive" (p. 90), and "selective and sensitive" (p. 92).

Audio and video recordings of counselling conversations have generally been made for education, training, assessment, and supervision purposes. In these circumstances, the direct benefit is seen to be primarily for the counsellor or student counsellor, who will use the tape for developmental, accountability or credentialing purposes. Clearly, a further hope is that current and future clients benefit from the learning that ensues when counsellors review recordings of their practice. Some counsellors also use video-recording as a therapeutic intervention – for example, reviewing tapes with clients in subsequent sessions, in a collaborative spirit of shared consultation (Depree, 2009).

In putting to work counselling values and ethical principles, counsellors might take into account the following guidelines, in particular, when they engage in electronic recording.

Competence Since reviewing practice contributes to counsellor accountability and thereby enhances our practice, throughout our professional lives, electronic recording can make a substantial contribution to the ongoing development of competence. However, before inviting clients (or other counselling students) to participate in recording, we should consider our competence, in terms of:

- using the technology itself;
- anticipating and responding appropriately to any anxieties we experience in relation with our own performances as counsellors so that we attend fully to the client and our facilitation of the counselling process.

We should have clarity ourselves about the purpose for which we are recording, and the time frame for retaining or erasing electronic recordings.

Informed consent Counsellors should give clients clear information about the use to be made of any recording – whether it is for the counsellor's self-review, for supervision, assessment or research purposes – and the request should be made in such a way that clients can decline as readily as they can agree to this request. Supervisors, teachers or classmates who will hear or view the recording should be named as part of an informed consent process, unless a recording is made for a wider audience. If the latter is intended, counsellors should describe clearly the nature, extent and limits of prospective audiences.

Professional disclosure statements Given to clients at the outset of therapy, these can assist in preparing clients for a possible request to record electronically. Clients should be informed that it is possible to change their mind about recording, even if they have initially agreed; to turn off the recording at any point; or to change their mind after a recording has been made but before it has been viewed. Verbal requests and explanations should be accompanied by written information about the purpose of the recording, and client consent should be recorded in writing. Some counsellors prefer a two-stage consent process – one before the recording, and a second once the recording has been made. At the time of this second consent, a client might choose, for example, that only a particular part of the recording is seen by others, or that a transcript is made but the visual recording is not used.

Storage and confidentiality Electronic recordings should be stored with the same concern for privacy as any other counselling records/notes (see Carol White, Part 3, Section 2). It is important that electronic storage is password protected (see Jeannie Wright, Part 3, Section 14). Recordings should be erased once the purpose for which they were made has been served, and in any case there should be an agreed time limit. Permanent erasure of electronic recordings from computers is a complex procedure, and seeking expert technical advice is strongly recommended.

Because recorded material could be required by a Court of law or a disciplinary body, it is important to exercise discretion about retaining recordings that contain particularly sensitive material.

What if a client asks to record or for a copy of a recording? I have found it useful to discuss with clients how they propose to use recordings, to guard against possible harm and to enhance the possibility of benefit. Again, I think it is useful to make a written agreement about this so that it is clear that our purposes are mutually understood. A counsellor should encourage clients, too, for their own safety and privacy, to consider appropriate storage, as they would with any other personal materials.

Responding to individual or cultural preferences New technologies are more available and familiar in some contexts than others, and we should act with care and respect for individual and cultural differences. For example, when it might be inappropriate for a client's face to be seen, the placing of a camera can be negotiated. Cultural consultation may also contribute to a counsellor's competence in particular situations, where recording is less familiar.

The NZAC National Newsletter has offered a forum, over a number of years, for discussion of benefits and cautions in audio and video recording. Of the cautions discussed there, one that has particularly stayed with me was George Sweet's suggestion that those whose counselling is made public through recording are likely to be "disadvantaged" (1998, p. 27). His caution offers a reminder to ensure that requests to record counselling conversations are made equitably, both in terms of what recording asks of clients, and what it might give them access to.

Recording supervision Supervisors and practitioners should traverse similar ethical considerations in recording supervision conversations. Such recordings might be made for a number of purposes – for later review by counsellors to enhance their learning, for a supervisor's professional development, or for a counsellor to take a purposefully recorded supervision conversation back to a client (see Crocket, 2004).

"Taking it back practices" (White, 1997, p. 142) While some practitioners have expressed concern that using taping for credentialing purposes benefits only the counsellor, others employ practices that offer clients some kind of response from those, particularly supervisors, who have

listened to or viewed a recording (see Crocket et al., 2009). White's (2007) outsider witness practices provide an ethically responsive map of such a practice.

FURTHER READING

The *Journal of Technology in Counseling* may be of interest to those with particular technical interests and expertise.

3.16
RESPONSIBILITIES TO OTHERS IN A CLIENT'S LIFE

Eric Medcalf, Margaret Agee, Sue Cornforth and Kathie Crocket

The centrality of partnership in the NZAC *Code of Ethics* (2002) highlights that the relational dimensions of counselling extend beyond the immediate counsellor–client relationship towards wider social networks. This section emphasises counsellors' responsibilities to others in clients' lives, particularly those to whom clients are emotionally connected.

The *Code of Ethics* invokes a responsibility to "promote the safety and well-being of individuals, families, communities, whanau, hapu and iwi." Guidelines in Section 5.2, "Respecting diversity and promoting social justice," provide more specific guidance as to how the core values might be enacted. Together these clauses provide a clear expectation that counsellors consider the wider implications of their behaviour, including who else might benefit or be harmed in the course of their work with a client or clients.

There is perhaps a tension here: the historical roots of counselling theory in a Western humanistic/existentialist tradition, and the influential tradition of the medical model, have tended to produce the individual as the primary social unit. However, a focus on partnership invites a critical attitude to ideas and practices that take for granted the privileging of the individual that is implicit in this history. The importance of consideration of others in a client's life applies, whether a client overtly identifies with a communally oriented world view, or whether a client's cultural history is more influenced by individualism. What is at stake is a counsellor's moral responsibility for the relational contexts of clients' lives.

This kind of moral responsibility has traditionally been neglected in therapy, suggested Doherty (1995), an over-emphasis on individual self-interest "giving short shrift to family and community responsibilities" (p. 7). Arguing for therapists to consider moral questions in their work and to raise these with clients, he warned clients to be "wary" of the following in a therapist:

- "The therapist discourages all use of moral language."
- "The therapist is quick to urge or support cutoffs from other family members."
- "The therapist sees only negatives in your family or spouse."
- "The therapist always portrays you as the victim of others, not as someone who can also harm others."
- "The therapist disparages your sense of duty towards others." (pp. 183–5)

An example of the absence of relational consideration was provided by Crocket's (2005) critique of Holloway's (1995) description of a supervision intervention. With very little information, a supervisor told a student counsellor that her client was facing a developmental difficulty in leaving home, and that counselling should have a developmental focus to support the client to separate from her parents. There was no consideration given to the cultural or other appropriateness of such advice and whether it was in the client's or her family's interest for her to leave home.

Other examples of the importance of contextual relational consideration come to mind. When a client is moving out of a marriage in which there are children, effective counselling processes will involve supporting that client to consider how they might leave in a way that would reduce potential deleterious effects for the children. Most situations that clients bring to counselling have relational consequences: leaving a job, coming out as gay or lesbian, making a complaint against a perpetrator of sexual abuse. Such life events can produce unintended disruptions to relationships, including with third parties who are not in a direct professional relationship with the counsellor. Whatever our chosen practice orientation, it is a counsellor's responsibility to invite clients, with care, into conversations that consider the well-being of others, along with the well-being of the client.

THIRD PARTY GRIEVANCE

Occasionally affected third parties may feel aggrieved by a client's actions, and may seek to blame a counsellor or seek redress. At worst there may be a complaint to the counsellor's professional body, and the Health and Disability Commissioner. Of course a counsellor's defence to a complaint may well be that a practitioner is not responsible for the actions of a client and that good counselling will enable a client to reach their own conclusions, rather than to be advised or instructed by the counsellor. A sense of grievance may be inevitable. A counsellor must be able to account for their role and actions in the situation. They can do this by being able to speak about their efforts to bring out an awareness of the consequences of a client's actions on those who are affected by the actions.

In addition to these relational concerns, there is a further pragmatic value in taking account of third parties. In the case of a complaint, a counsellor is limited in their ability to defend themselves directly to a third party. A third party complainant is not a direct client. A counsellor has a duty of confidentiality towards the client and is bound by the contractual relationship with the client. Yet, any client may speak freely about the counselling and the counsellor. For example, a complainant may claim that the client said, "My counsellor said that you are ..." which could be anything from "bad for me" to "suffering from a personality disorder." Or, there may be an implication that the counsellor advised the client to take particular actions. These are complex situations for counsellors to negotiate, in consultation with supervisors.

THIRD PARTIES AND COUNSELLOR VULNERABILITIES AND BIASES

Counselling is a complex relational process and it is important that counsellors consider how their own life experiences, values, vulnerabilities and biases position them in relation to third parties. While it is possible to fail to consider third parties, it is also possible to over-identify with them. In either situation the effect may be that clients are not supported in their consideration of others in their lives. It is an important skill to discern between caring solidarity in standing alongside others (Sevenhuijsen, 1998), and unconsidered collusion.

Counsellors, their clients and third parties will benefit from a counsellor's mindfulness of the range of their relational responsibilities and willingness to consult in supervision, or in personal counselling. In considering the implications for others, counsellors contribute to positive outcomes for their clients and those close to them. While Fisher (2009) wrote about psychologists, her questions transfer into counselling.

> If we stop asking "Who is the client?" what should we ask instead? Regardless of the type of case or the number of relationships it involves, the question psychologists should ask might be "What exactly are my ethical responsibilities to each of the parties in this case?" (p. 5)

3.17
IMMINENT THREAT OF SERIOUS HARM

Margaret Agee

One of the most stressful circumstances in counselling practice occurs when there appears to be "imminent threat of serious harm" to a client or to others associated with a client (NZAC, 2002, 5.1.d). While this phrase is normally associated with indications of immediate or foreseeable suicidal or homicidal behaviour, it may also apply in a limited range of other circumstances. Most counsellors in New Zealand, according to Agee's (2001) survey of members of NZAC, have worked with suicidal clients, and have expressed confidence that their professional preparation and supervision equips them and supports them in this aspect of their practice. However, working to minimise risk can be highly demanding, involving multiple considerations in making what can be life or death decisions (Bond, 2010; Corey, Corey & Callanan, 2007). Maintaining competence and building effective collegial support in this area of practice is therefore crucial in ensuring that counsellors have well-established resources to draw on when working to support clients experiencing particular vulnerability.

Despite current knowledge about suicide and the factors that influence both vulnerability and resilience, predicting suicidal behaviour by individual clients is often very difficult (Ministry of Health, 2008a, 2008b). It is also difficult to evaluate the likelihood that a client will harm others. On one hand every threat needs to be taken seriously, but on the other, counsellors' professional judgement is called upon when determining how at-risk a particular client may be and how competent a client is to make decisions. Whether there is "serious danger in the immediate or foreseeable future" needs to be ascertained in context "on a case by case basis" (see Simon Jefferson, Part 4, Section 1).

Counsellors are required to exercise professional responsibility in making assessments, taking account of the contexts of a client's life and of the counsellor's professional setting. It is important that counsellors are involved in the development of agency or school practice guidelines, so that they are well positioned to make wise ethical decisions, situation by situation. While it is wise to err on the side of caution in order to avoid harm, care and caution should also be applied in taking any preventive action. Granello (2010) wrote of "a sort of therapeutic tunnel vision" (p. 363) that can produce a mechanical, anxiety-driven form of risk-assessment, de-contextualised from the therapeutic relationship. Enacting the value of responsible care (3.4) involves honouring the importance of both safety and therapeutic process.

Ethical dilemmas may not arise if a trusting relationship between counsellor and client is established, enabling that all steps to ensure a client's safety – including the involvement of selected others – are undertaken with the client's full knowledge and consent. If necessary, taking "all reasonable steps to protect clients from harm" (5.1. a), or warning "third parties and appropriate authorities" of potential imminent danger to a third party (5.1.d), may involve contravening a client's expressed wishes at a particular time. In so doing, a counsellor would be acting in accordance with the contractual agreement made at the beginning of the counselling relationship, to uphold the ethical obligation to protect the client's or others' lives. If no such contract had been made, by involving others a counsellor would still be acting in accordance with the NZAC *Code of Ethics*; action which can be framed positively within the counselling relationship as drawing on all the resources possible to help keep the client alive (Shallcross, 2010).

Because of the potential consequences, virtually all ethical guidelines among the helping professions, including the NZAC *Code of Ethics*, absolve practitioners of the duty to maintain client confidentiality in such situations, in order to reduce risk (6.2. a). The NZAC *Code of Ethics* states thus: "Exceptions to confidentiality occur when there is serious danger in the immediate or foreseeable future to the client or others" (6.2.c).

The second exception the Code lists – when a "client's competence to make a decision is impaired" (6.2.c) – could also be relevant in a life and death situation, when a client's reasoning is severely affected by emotional anguish, mental illness and/or by drugs or alcohol.

Underpinning these provisions is a moral responsibility to preserve life, expressed through the core value of responsible caring (3.4), and the ethical principle to promote the safety and well being of individuals, families, communities, whānau, hapū and iwi (4.5).

This imperative can require counsellors to address tensions between core values – of autonomy (3.3), and responsible caring (3.4) – as well as between ethical principles promoting safety (4.5) and respecting confidences (4.4). The question of ultimate client autonomy over life and death decisions is controversial, as well as complex, presenting both practical and ethical challenges (Bond, 2010). These challenges call on counsellors' professional knowledge, judgement and wisdom in order to respond effectively "with care and respect for individual and cultural differences" (4.1), in ways that "avoid doing harm" (4.2), are "honest and trustworthy" (4.6), and involve "practice within the scope of their competence" (4.7).

Because of the exceptional nature of these situations in which exceptions to confidentiality may be exercised, the NZAC *Code of Ethics* gives more detailed guidance regarding the processes to follow. The *Code* cautions practitioners to pass on "only the minimum of information necessary and only then to those people to whom it is absolutely necessary" (6.2.b). It advises counsellors, if possible, to seek the client's cooperation before breaking confidentiality, "unless doing so would further compromise the safety of the client or others" (6.2.d), as well as consulting with a supervisor or senior colleague, before acting.

When there is potential for suicide, sensitive discernment is necessary so that the involvement of others reduces rather than exacerbates the risk of harm. For example, serious difficulties in relationships with close family members may be a contributing factor to a client's distress. Other sources of support may need to be found in the immediate crisis; and part of the ongoing work of counselling may involve restoration of relationship between the client and parents, partner or the wider family.

In a crisis involving imminent risk of harm, accessing effective external support for clients from mental health, statutory and community agencies involves counsellors in liaison, referral and advocacy. Ethical guidelines regarding referral (5.14) and relationships with other professionals (7.4), and the ethical principle of responsible care therefore also apply in these circumstances. Responsible caring involves not only effective action when imminent danger of serious harm becomes apparent, but also involves longer term work, building relationships with other professionals in relevant external agencies and services over time. In this way, the foundations are laid for effective collaboration when it is needed most, in order to promote safety.

PART 4

ETHICS AND THE LAW

4.1 ETHICS AND THE LAW

Simon Jefferson

INTRODUCTION

In addition to ethical obligations, a counsellor has legal obligations. However, the interface between the law and the ethics of counselling is not always smooth. Counselling is a client-centred process in which experiences are explored and examined in a collaborative fashion. It is quintessentially a voluntary process, built on a relationship of trust between a counsellor and a client. That relationship is both contractual and fiduciary, and thus generates a series of mutual obligations that are both ethical in substance and enforceable, on occasions, under the law.

Since Rogers' (1962) seminal work, empathy, sensitivity and a suspension of judgement have been qualities that characterise counsellors and inform the counselling process. Counselling is founded on an intention to compassionately understand the other.

By comparison, the law is a rather more brutal beast, judgemental by definition and certainly less nuanced in its processes. Unlike counselling, the law is designed to meet the needs of the broader community, not the individual, and the maintenance of the rule of law is a key constitutional objective of the State.

Inevitably the existence of external, legal constraints will pose continuing challenges and dilemmas for counsellors.

Some of the constraints imposed by the law are clearly in step with the ethical requirements which counsellors in New Zealand, generally through the NZAC *Code of Ethics*, impose upon themselves. For example, substantive obligations imposed under the Fair Trading Act 1986 (constraining a counsellor from claiming qualifications or experience unjustifiably), the Consumer Guarantees Act 1993 (requiring anyone providing a service to ensure that it is carried out with reasonable care and skill) and the Medicines Act 1981 (making it an offence to publish untrue advertisements in relation to therapeutic treatments), are no greater than the obligations which can be found in the *Code of Ethics,* although they will carry with them state-imposed penalties for breach and even, in some circumstances, a risk of prosecution.

In a more general sense, there are constraints imposed upon counsellors which are imposed on every other New Zealander, but which may have ramifications in terms of practice. For example, counsellors must refrain from committing acts of discrimination in terms of the Human Rights Act 1993.

Finally, there are constraints, such as those imposed by the Privacy Act 1993 in relation to collection, use, disclosure and storage of personal information. In practical terms these may amount to little more than sound business and administrative practice. For example, the obligation to retain counselling records in secure storage would not only meet the requirements of the Privacy Act 1993, but also the ethical obligations imposed by the *Code of Ethics* (NZAC, 2002). However, some counsellors continue to struggle with meeting the standards set by the Privacy Act 1993, and, by failing to meet those standards – for example, in note-taking practices – they expose themselves not only to the strictures of the Privacy Act 1993, but also to allegations of professional misconduct, in terms of the *Code of Ethics.*

It is understandable that, faced with the mysteries and complexities of the law, counsellors may experience anxiety. How, for example, does a counsellor reconcile the need to take notes with the potential that, one day, those notes may be required as evidence in a court of law? That raises questions not only of the extent and nature of the note taking, but also the period for which such notes should be retained. Medcalf (see Part 3, Section 1) suggests that pursuant to the Health (Retention of Health Information) Regulations 1996, such notes must be kept for a minimum of 10 years. Non-compliance renders a counsellor vulnerable to prosecution and a fine.

THE STATUS OF CODES OF ETHICS

It is important to note that a code of ethics is not a legal document, but an internally generated set of professional guidelines. Codes of ethics can, and frequently will, be modified and amended to respond to contemporary understanding of professional issues. At any given time, a code of ethics will constitute the collective wisdom of the professional body which has generated it and an accumulation of best practice standards. More often than not, codes of ethics are expressed in general terms. They are not designed to cover every eventuality and do not, of themselves, provide penalties for non-compliance.

Generally, membership of a professional body such as the New Zealand Association of Counsellors will carry with it an obligation to subscribe and adhere to that body's code of ethics. Members of a professional body may find their professional conduct measured, by that body, against the code of ethics in the course of internal disciplinary proceedings. In the event that the professional conduct of a member also becomes the subject of court proceedings, a court is likely to take into account the code of ethics as representing the single most important indicator of what does or does not constitute a lack of appropriate skill and care. It should be noted, however, that a code of ethics is not necessarily the only, or the determinative indicator, of appropriate skill and care.

COUNSELLORS AND LEGAL OBLIGATIONS

The source of a counsellor's legal obligation may be statutory (by virtue of an Act of Parliament or Statutory Regulation), arise from the operation of common law (being the accretion of custom and jurisprudence) or, increasingly, derive from New Zealand's obligations under various international covenants and treaties to which it has acceded (for example, United Nations Convention on the Rights of the Child).

In its simplest form the law in New Zealand can be discerned from an analysis of Acts of Parliament and Statutory Regulations promulgated by Parliament. Many of the statutory instruments refer directly to counsellors and the profession generally. The creation of the Family Court in 1981, embracing a multi-disciplinary model in which counselling and mediation were seen as integral parts of the Family Court process, saw the enactment of the Family Proceedings Act 1980. A number of other current Acts of Parliament are also relevant to counselling, including:

- Contraception, Sterilisation and Abortion Act 1977;
- Adult Adoption Information Act 1985;
- Children Young Persons and Their Families Act 1989;
- Education Act 1989;

- Victim Rights Act 2002;
- Health Practitioners Competence Assurance Act 2003.

Other statutes are of more general application but impact directly upon the profession of counselling.

In most instances, a counsellor's ethical obligations will run in parallel with those legal obligations, but on occasion conflicts, or apparent conflicts, do arise. In such circumstances, a counsellor's legal obligations will invariably prevail. In that sense, in New Zealand counselling is not a privileged occupation. Confidentiality, in particular, is an ethical practice, not a legal right authorised by statute.

CONFIDENTIALITY, PRIVILEGE AND ITS LIMITS

It is important to distinguish between the ethic of confidentiality and the legal concept of confidentiality, more accurately called *privilege*. In essence, privilege is an extension of confidentiality.

Confidentiality is at the heart of the counsellor–client relationship and comprises a duty, owed by the counsellor, not to disclose, without the client's informed consent, communications made by the client during the course of that relationship.

Questions of privilege arise when a counsellor is asked to disclose to a court, a judicial body, or a quasi-judicial body, what would be confidential information in the context of the counsellor–client relationship. A quasi-judicial body is a body created by statute and charged with decision-making. The Human Rights Tribunal, the Employment Tribunal and the Disputes Tribunal are examples. Information which may be required to be disclosed to such a body may be in the form of written documentation or oral testimony.

In such circumstances, disclosure of relevant information is, as a general proposition, regarded as beneficial, and any exception to that has to be justified as serving a greater public interest. This is because the effect of a successful claim of privilege (that is, a right of non disclosure) is to ensure that relevant information is withheld from the Court and cannot be brought into account in the decision-making process. Thus there is obvious moral competition between, on one hand, the legal importance of all relevant information being made available to a tribunal to ensure that justice is done, and, on the other hand, the social importance of upholding, preserving and encouraging certain confidential relationships. It follows, therefore, that the law has been reluctant to extend too widely the ability to claim privilege. Some good cause, plainly shown, is required to establish the existence of any privilege. The crucial question is whether the interest sought to be protected by the claim of privilege (the confidential counsellor–client relationship) is at least as important as the proper administration of justice. Any endeavour to withhold relevant evidence under a claim of privilege will be carefully, even jealously, scrutinised in judicial settings.

Privilege, in its legal sense, is a special right, advantage, or immunity granted to a particular group. Thus parliamentary privilege protects members of Parliament from legal liability for statements made during parliamentary debates. The underlying principle is plain: it is considered that the greater benefit to society is in permitting free discourse within Parliament, rather than in inhibiting freedom of speech to protect the reputation of individuals. Similarly, no witness giving testimony in a court case – whether orally or by way of affidavit – can be subjected to civil proceedings at the suit of someone who considers they have been wronged or defamed by such evidence. Historically, and perhaps quaintly in 21st century New Zealand, three professions hold an exalted status in the context of privilege – lawyers, doctors and priests. The scope of that privilege is not perhaps as great as it once was, but, equally, the categories of those professions entitled to claim *absolute privilege* has not been expanded to embrace other groups who, in contemporary society, might well be seen as performing at least as vital a role in providing assistance to members of the community, the so-called helping professions.

Thus, it is important to note that the ethical obligation upon a counsellor to maintain confidentiality does not automatically translate into a legal right to refuse to disclose information under specific circumstances. In the context of court proceedings, whether criminal or civil, it is well established that a witness must, and is under a compulsion to, give information relevant to the proceedings, unless the Court holds otherwise on grounds of public policy or unless the witness is entitled to claim privilege whether pursuant to statute or otherwise.

For example, a witness may properly decline to answer questions because the answers would, or might, give rise to the risk of criminal proceedings (but not because the answers would, or might, expose the witness to the risk of a civil claim or disciplinary proceedings). This is known as the privilege against self-incrimination. Other examples are unlikely to have much immediate relevance to counsellors: a married witness can refuse to disclose spousal communications made during the marriage (in Massachusetts efforts have been made to extend that to parent–child communications); certain communications between lawyers and clients, doctors and patients, and priests and penitents, are also privileged with the right to waive privilege resting with the client, patient or penitent. In the ordinary course of events, a counsellor called to give evidence in court proceedings is deemed to be a compellable witness, and, on the face of it, has no greater right than any other citizen to decline to answer relevant questions properly asked. The shield of confidentiality inherent in the counselling relationship will not, of itself, afford the counsellor protection.

STATUTORY PROTECTION FOR COUNSELLORS

A counsellor does have some statutory protections. A counsellor carrying out functions under the Family Proceedings Act 1980 (counselling in the Family Court context) is protected by an absolute prohibition concerning the giving of evidence of any information, statements or admissions disclosed or made in the course of such counselling (section 18, Family Proceedings Act 1980). Similar provisions may be found in the Children Young Persons and Their Families Act 1989 and the Domestic Violence Act 1995. These provisions not only preclude the clients themselves giving evidence of information, statements or admissions disclosed in the course of counselling, but also prohibit counsellors from doing so. However, this protection is strictly limited to those counsellors carrying out functions pursuant to Part II, Family Proceedings Act 1980, and does not extend to counsellors carrying out functions as a private counsellor, even though this may be in the context of marital counselling or Family Court proceedings. However, over and beyond that absolute prohibition, there is a statutory provision of which a counsellor may seek to avail him/herself. Pursuant to that provision, a witness may seek to be excused from answering all or any questions asked in the course of court proceedings. The court, faced with such a request, has a discretion to excuse a witness from answering questions. The exercise of that discretion, on a case-by-case basis, is essentially informed by the need to balance the importance of encouraging and preserving the special relationship existing between counsellor and client with a public interest in having the information disclosed.

A recent statutory provision sets out in a clear and easy fashion the basic fact that, in any situation involving the disclosure of confidential communications or information to public interests, consideration needs to be given to section 69, Evidence Act 2006. These considerations and balance refer to:

a. the public interest in the disclosure of the particular communications or information;

b. the public interest in preserving confidences in relationships, and disclosures made on the basis of those confidences.

Section 69 of the Evidence Act 2006 sets out a series of matters which need to be brought into account in carrying out this balancing exercise:

a. The nature of any harm which might be occasioned by the disclosure;

b. The nature of the confidential material and its importance to the proceeding then before the Court;

c. The nature of the proceedings;

d. Whether there are other means of getting the information before the Court;

e. Whether the information can be brought before the Court in such a way as to restrict its disclosure, given the sensitivity of the information and given the time elapsed in any other disclosure made.

DISCLOSURE OF DOCUMENTATION

It is not only the giving of oral testimony which raises issues of confidentiality. Disclosure of documentation in the preparatory legal process (known as *discovery*) can also prove vexing. In 1998 the matter was considered by the New Zealand Court of Appeal where the issue before the Court was whether or not notes made by doctors and counsellors consulted by the plaintiffs in some civil proceedings were to be *privileged from disclosure.* More specifically, the issue was whether or not, following discovery of the notes by the plaintiffs, the defendants were entitled to an order enabling them to inspect these documents. To understand the outcome of the Court of Appeal's decision, it is important to distinguish between the process of *discovery,* in which acknowledgement of the existence of various documents is required, and *inspection,* in which the party to whom the existence of the documents has been disclosed seeks to view those documents. Perhaps not surprisingly, the judicial instinct is for disclosure as opposed to suppression. It is a serious step to exclude evidence relevant to an issue, because it is in the public interests that the search for truth should, in general, be unfettered. Broadly speaking, the same considerations as apply to a request to be excused from giving oral testimony will apply. On that basis the issue will tend to be dealt with on a case-by-case basis.

DUTY TO WARN

A concept familiar to most counsellors is the so-called *duty to warn* (NZAC, 2002) which provides an exception to the obligation of confidentiality attached to counsellor–client relationships. In such cases, a counsellor has, in effect, a discretion to disclose what would otherwise be confidential, since protecting safety and well-being (4.5) take precedence over respecting confidences (4.4). (See Margaret Agee, Part 3, Section 17, for further discussion of this point.) Of course, when we have already clarified the limits of confidentiality as part of informed consent processes, such disclosure does not constitute a breach of confidentiality, in any case.

The most obvious statutory manifestation, in New Zealand, of the duty to warn is found in Children Young Persons and Their Families Act 1989, section 15. Pursuant to that section, any person who believes that any child or young person has been, or is likely to be, harmed, whether physically, emotionally or sexually, ill-treated, abused, neglected, or deprived, may report the matter to a social worker (in effect a social worker employed by Child Youth and Family Services) or to the Police, without fear of being subject subsequently to civil, criminal, or disciplinary procedures, provided that the disclosure of the information is made in good faith.

Outside the paradigm of the Children Young Persons and Their Families Act 1989, counsellors retain an entitlement to act outside of the ethic of counsellor–client confidentiality where it is considered that there is a serious and imminent risk that the client will cause harm to him/herself or to some other party. The most frequently cited legal basis for this duty to warn is the Californian case of Tarasoff v The Regents of the University of California 551P.2d 334 (1976). Whilst that decision was given in the context of a claim for damages for negligence – a context which is unlikely to arise in the New Zealand legal system – it nevertheless has provided a useful outline of the limits on client–counsellor confidentiality.

Consideration of the *duty to warn* raises a number of significant issues.

- What is confidential information? A search for a definition of this has proved surprisingly elusive, and has tended to be dealt with on a pragmatic basis. Communications may be identified as confidential either because of the nature of the information itself or because of the circumstances in which it is communicated.
- Is the duty to warn a positive duty or simply permissive? Concepts of best practice would suggest that whilst the imposition of a positive duty to warn goes further than the law requires, it is likely that a failure to warn in some circumstances may well amount to an action falling below the relevant standards of professionalism.
- What is "imminent threat of serious harm" (NZAC, 2002) or serious risk of harm? Inevitably, and perhaps unhelpfully, this is always going to be a matter of judgement to be considered on a case-by-case basis. For further discussion see Margaret Agee (Part 3, Section 17).
- To whom should disclosure be made? The NZAC *Code of Ethics* says that a counsellor should warn both third parties and appropriate authorities (5.1.d) when there is imminent threat of serious harm to third parties. In other situations, such as where there appears to be risk to the safety of children, questions of whether disclosure should be made to authorities constitute another judgement for the counsellor to make, in consultation with agency policies and protocols.
- Should an intention to disclose be notified, in advance, to the client? Again, this may be a question of the nature of the "harm" and the "risk" which has been identified. The potential risk in notifying a client in advance should be carefully assessed: there will be times when responsible care will involve taking actions without notifying a client in order to protect the safety of others or of a counsellor themselves.

A counsellor will inevitably wrestle with a significant dilemma when confronted with circumstances in which the duty to warn may arise, and, on balance, a conservative approach, erring towards disclosure rather than confidentiality, is likely to be justifiable. Consultation with supervisors or senior and trusted colleagues is always appropriate in such situations.

QUESTIONS TO ASK IN PREPARING FOR COURT

Counsellors are increasingly called upon to give evidence in court. This can be in civil proceedings (see for example G v G (1996) 15FRNZ 22), criminal proceedings, or, increasingly frequently, Family Court proceedings.

Courts can be daunting arenas, operating within a paradigm quite foreign to most counsellors, and in many respects quite contrary to a counselling ethos. Even within the Family Court, the essential model remains adversarial and the question–answer format, coupled with formal protocols and rules of procedure, can feel quite stilted and awkward. Whether or not such a process is the best means of achieving the stated goals – the ascertaining of truth, the determination of the best interests of the child, and justice – may be the subject of much debate, but for a counsellor appearing in court, it is important to recognise and work in terms of the process as it is.

Counsellors requested to give evidence in court proceedings should take into account the following:

- Has the client authorised the giving of evidence or even authorised a discussion with a lawyer or prosecuting authority about the possibility of giving evidence?
- Is the counsellor inhibited or prohibited by law (for example section 18 Family Proceedings Act 1980) from giving the evidence sought, in any event?
- Even if there is no statutory inhibition does the counsellor, in the circumstances, consider that there is a basis for asking to be excused from giving evidence?
- Who is requesting that the evidence be given? For example, in proceedings under the Care of Children Act 2004 it is frequently unwise and even unprofessional to be inveigled by one adult party or the other to give testimony. It would be naïve not to appreciate that evidence coming from a professional, qualified, counsellor is being placed before the Court to give additional weight by virtue of presumed or assumed professional expertise.
- Is the evidence being sought to be adduced *observational* (that is, what a counsellor saw or heard) or *expert*? If expert evidence is being sought, does a counsellor, in fact, have the necessary and requisite expertise to qualify as an expert witness? This is a

question of competence (5.9.c). A counsellor should take care to distinguish between *observational* evidence and *expert* evidence, a distinction those seeking evidence might blur.

- If a counsellor is requested to give *expert* opinion evidence, is the counsellor able to substantiate the opinions, from reputable and reliable sources? Is a counsellor sufficiently objective and independent to act properly as an expert witness?

Above all, in giving evidence in court proceedings, anything said by a witness – whether observational or expert – will inevitably form part, and part only, of the evidential jigsaw.

It is therefore important that counsellors, in giving evidence, distinguish between professional input and advocacy for or on behalf of one party or the other, or on behalf of the child. Again, the counsellor's code of ethics must cede ground to the formalities of the court process. Traversing these paradigmatically different domains – courtrooms and counselling rooms – may be a difficult process and counsellors are advised to maintain their competence through this process through regular supervision (5.9.a).

Where a counsellor has been asked to give evidence, it is of considerable importance that the counsellor is properly briefed by the lawyer who is calling the evidence. It is inappropriate to be asked to simply attend court on a given day, at a given time. Any witness is entitled to clarify the nature of the evidence to be given, to ensure that the evidence being given is indeed relevant to the matters in issue before the Court, and to be prepared for the sort of questions which may be posed under cross examination or indeed by a judge. Assisting a witness in this way is an essential part of the lawyer's tasks. Counsellors should not be timid in asking the lawyer for that sort of assistance. In addition, an explanation of the process and procedure should be sought.

4.2
COUNSELLORS AS WITNESSES IN COURT

Margaret Agee and Rachael Feather

Whereas once it was a rare occurrence, it is now increasingly likely that counsellors will be asked to give evidence in court (see Simon Jefferson, Part 4, Section 1) or in quasi-judicial proceedings. In some circumstances, such as a situation in which a counsellor has been the first person to whom a child has disclosed abuse, and the perpetrator is prosecuted, the counsellor will almost inevitably be called upon for testimony. In other circumstances, a request from a client or a client's legal representative to give evidence will present an ethical dilemma that challenges a counsellor to consider the course of action that will be in the best interests of the client. Thirdly, local research suggests that practitioners may be just as likely to testify voluntarily as they are to testify at the request of the Court (Feather & Agee, 2000).

In the second and third of these circumstances, the desire to help a client through providing testimony or acting as an observational witness can be compelling. To do so may seem to be acting in accordance with the core values in the NZAC *Code of Ethics* of responsible caring (3.4) and social justice (3.6; 5.1.b; 5.2.f). If the case concerned domestic violence or sexual abuse the principle of safety (4.5) would be relevant. At the same time it has been suggested that counsellors may at times too willingly become involved in clients' legal issues (Remley, 1991). Counsellors who have acted as witnesses have reported feeling highly ambivalent and have experienced conflict throughout their participation in the legal process, and have found the experience extremely stressful both professionally and personally (Feather & Agee, 2000).

In addition, as Simon Jefferson (Part 4, Section 1) has pointed out, counsellors may also be at ethical risk of practising beyond the scope of their competence if they agree to testify as expert witnesses to matters in which they do not in fact have sufficient expertise. However, the risks of practising outside the boundaries of their competence, as well as of doing harm to clients, to their own reputations, and to the standing of the profession, are also present if counsellors testify as observational witnesses without having considered the full consequences of doing so, and without adequate preparation. These consequences may include, but are not limited to: building unrealistic expectations in clients; becoming involved when a counsellor has little to contribute or may in fact harm a client's case; letting a client down as a result of acquitting oneself poorly, thereby damaging the therapeutic relationship; and/ or experiencing the effects of trauma both during and for some time after the legal proceedings have concluded, which can impair a counsellor's capacity to practise effectively.

In view of these concerns, it seems particularly important to engage in a thorough, well-informed ethical and practical decision-making process in order to formulate a considered and wise response to any request or opportunity to give evidence in legal proceedings. Part 1, Section 5 of this book offers one of many useful frameworks. In making a decision about a request or opportunity to provide testimony, the considerations outlined in Part 1, Section 5 play a vital role in guiding practitioners' thinking and information seeking, in addition to consulting the NZAC *Code of Ethics* and other resources or consultants relevant to the situation. Seeking legal advice (6.3.a) that is independent of a client's legal adviser is always recommended for a counsellor's own protection, in advance of any involvement in legal proceedings. Depending upon the terms of particular insurance policies, counsellors who hold professional indemnity insurance can access advice free of charge from specified legal practitioners. Situations have also arisen in which counsellors have needed to seek advice from an independent source other than their agency or organisation's legal adviser. An employer's lawyer has no legal obligation to a counsellor, whose interests may not be consistent with those of the employer; furthermore, this discrepancy may not become apparent until proceedings are already underway.

When counsellors are to testify in legal proceedings, careful preparation is needed in order to practise with competence in an unfamiliar environment, governed by different values, rules and conventions from those of the counselling world. Professional responsibility and personal fear sit uneasily alongside each other; even experienced practitioners may find themselves relatively powerless in a personally threatening situation. The challenge is therefore "to equip oneself as best as possible to function competently in that foreign context" (Feather & Agee, 2000, p. 59). Responsible preparation involves: first seeking supervision with an appropriately resourced supervisor; recognising where preparation is needed, and identifying appropriate sources of assistance; gaining a fundamental understanding of the legal system; seeking information about what to expect regarding courtroom procedures; understanding what is expected of the witness role; and instruction or coaching in handling questioning processes, particularly in responding to challenging cross-examination.

Alongside the practical preparation it is important to anticipate the emotional effects of courtroom experience. Counsellors have found it helpful to set up personal and professional support for the courtroom experience and afterwards, including the preparation of friends and family, and to have someone present in the courtroom to offer emotional support, to bear witness to what transpired, and to debrief with afterwards (Feather & Agee, 2000). Supervisors have a substantial role in supporting counsellors through every aspect of legal processes, including helping practitioners navigate their way through decision-making processes, helping them identify and access sources of information and advice, as well as facilitating debriefing and support after testifying. Counsellors need to feel free to ask their supervisors about their knowledge in this area, and may need to seek additional support from another supervisor with experience of these processes.

Counsellors are also caring responsibly when they explore with clients the implications of their involvement in their court proceedings for their relationship and their ongoing work together. Such exploration includes:

- involving clients in the initial decision-making process if possible, and also talking about expectations;
- discussing with clients the differences between the culture of the counselling room and the courtroom, to minimise the discomfort that could ensue when meeting in the courtroom environment;
- helping prepare clients for what to expect in the courtroon environment, including personal reactions both client and counsellor might experience, and working out coping strategies;

- exploring what might be asked of the counsellor, including implications regarding the disclosure of client information, and the discomfort this could evoke, particularly if the Court requires disclosure that goes beyond what the client and the counsellor anticipate or would want;
- preparing clients for potentially disappointing as well as hoped-for outcomes so that they are as fully informed about the process as possible.

In these ways, the therapeutic relationship can be safeguarded as far as possible, and the potential for harm to clients as a result of the counsellor's involvement as a witness can be minimised.

4.3
WHEN A CLIENT GOES TO COURT

Margaret Agee

When clients become involved in legal or quasi-judicial proceedings, counsellors may face uncertainty regarding the most ethically appropriate ways in which to respond. Such situations may occur:

- when a client goes to court as a defendant in a criminal trial;
- when a client acts as a witness;
- when a client is involved in Family Court proceedings;
- when a client is subject to disciplinary action, such as a Board of Trustees hearing regarding potential suspension from school, or employment-related proceedings;
- or when a client or supervisee is a complainant or a respondent in a hearing.

Given the serious consequences that can be at stake for clients, and the unfamiliar and intimidating nature of such proceedings, counsellors can have a valuable part to play in helping them to prepare, and in providing psychological support throughout these processes.

WHEN A CLIENT CONSIDERS GOING TO COURT

Prior to this stage, counsellors may assist clients in making decisions about whether to take legal action against someone else, whether to lay a complaint through quasi-judicial channels, or whether to volunteer to act as a witness in a hearing. Reflecting the core value of social justice (3.6), the NZAC *Code of Ethics* (2002) declares: "Counsellors shall support their clients to challenge the injustices they experience." However, in particular situations, encouraging a client to pursue a complaint through formal channels or become otherwise involved in legal proceedings, may not be in that person's best interests. If a counsellor unquestioningly supports a client's decision to take formal action (3.3) or becomes persuasive and encourages the client to take action without full regard to the potential consequences, the practitioner may inadvertently do harm (5.1.a). Instead, responsible caring (3.4) involves ensuring that clients have considered all relevant factors, including potential consequences and alternative courses of action, and have consulted when necessary with legal or procedural advisers in making a fully informed decision.

ISSUES TO CONSIDER WHEN SUPPORTING A CLIENT GOING TO COURT

When a client has become involved in legal or quasi-judicial processes, providing empathic, psychological preparation and support may lead counsellors to overstep the boundaries of professional competence (4.7), and potentially do harm if, out of a desire to provide care, they offer information or suggestions that are beyond their expertise. Working "within the limits of their knowledge, training and experience" (5.9.c) adjures counsellors to refrain from giving legal advice, but involves working to ensure that clients are well represented and well briefed. This could include:

- engaging with or referral to others who have relevant expertise to help prepare the client;
- helping the client to access relevant written resources (Courts 128, 2009; Courts 129, 2009);
- ensuring the client is well represented, and liaising with lawyers on behalf of the client when necessary;
- and addressing other aspects of the client's support needs (Ludbrook, 2003).

If, however, a client is alleged to have committed a crime, or has committed a crime, or has taken an ambiguous role, or a role that seems at odds with the counsellor's values, conflict between personal reactions and professional duty may compromise a practitioner's capacity to maintain an effective therapeutic relationship with the client. It would be important to discuss the situation in supervision, and to consider referring the client to another practitioner who could provide effective support through the legal process (5.14.a).

ATTENDING A HEARING

Ethical conflicts can arise over the question of whether to attend a hearing as a support person or advocate for a client. It is commonly part of a school counsellor's role to ensure that students have adequate representation or advocacy at disciplinary hearings run by Boards of Trustees. The latter may be limited to writing a report in support of the client (Ludbrook, 2003), but some counsellors frequently attend these hearings in person.

Each situation is unique, and the ethical values and principles that guide counsellors in considering the appropriateness of attending any formal hearing as a support person for a client include the values of responsible caring and social justice, as well as the ethical principle of promoting the safety and well-being of individuals and communities (4.5). The protection of client information (4.4) may also be relevant.

Attending a hearing may require both careful thought on the part of a counsellor and sensitive negotiation with the client. Issues regarding acting as a witness in court are addressed in the preceding section of this book. If attendance involves a non-active support role in proceedings, factors that need to be considered include:

- fairness with regard to a practitioner's capacity to meet the client's needs alongside professional responsibilities to others;
- congruence with the value of responsible caring and minimal risk of harm to the client, or to the therapeutic relationship (4.2). For example, could attendance result in blurred role boundaries that could jeopardise the ongoing counselling relationship (5.11.c)? Or if shameful information not previously disclosed to the counsellor is revealed in a hearing, how might the counsellor act to minimise the risk of harm to the therapeutic relationship?
- maintenance of client privacy. If family members, friends, or associates of the client are likely to be present, what knowledge do they have of the counselling relationship? How will client and counsellor explain to others the counsellor's presence and role, and what risks might be entailed for the client or for the counsellor? The very existence of the therapeutic relationship may be deeply sensitive, constituting personal information that a client may need to protect (6.1).

For school counsellors, some situations can be particularly challenging, and involvement in student disciplinary processes and hearings can involve negotiating tensions between conflicting aspects of their role:

their duty to provide guidance and counselling in accordance with section 77(a) of the Education Act 1989 to individual students who are subject to suspension and stand-down (Ludbrook, 2003), including advocacy when necessary; and their accountability to colleagues and to the administration, as well as responsibility for the well-being of the school as a community. In helping counsellors manage role conflicts regarding their multiple accountabilities and the need to "clarify, adjust, or withdraw from these roles by an appropriate process" (5.11.h) if necessary, supervision is likely to play an important part.

Furthermore, while counsellors are encouraged in the NZAC *Code of Ethics* to "promote social justice through advocacy and empowerment" (5.2.h), becoming an advocate for a client through legal or quasi-judicial means should only be undertaken:

- after consultation with the client about this course of action and careful consideration together of the potential consequences;
- with the client's fully informed consent (5.5);
- when client and counsellor have established a clear and explicit contract about the action the practitioner is to take and any client information that may be disclosed to others by the counsellor.

Taking these steps helps ensure that a client maintains control over the nature and limits of personal information shared on his or her behalf, and also helps ensure that the pace of the process is consistent with the client's resources and capacity to cope.

4.4 WHEN A COUNSELLOR KNOWS ABOUT ILLEGAL PRACTICES

Margaret Agee

In day-to-day professional practice, holding confidences about clients' circumstances and life experiences can be emotionally demanding for counsellors. Hearing clients talk about illegal activities involving themselves and/or other people known to them can not only be particularly disturbing, but can also raise questions about a counsellor's wider responsibilities. Illegal activities may include: illegal use and/or sale of psychoactive substances; all forms of violence, including sexual abuse; buying and distributing alcohol while under the legal age; illegal gambling; theft; various forms of fraud; participating in the illegal, informal economy; and other offenses. Counsellors may hear of such activities in any practice setting, but they are perhaps more likely to do so when working in agencies dealing with problem gambling, alcohol and drug counselling, in schools, in community agencies, and in tertiary education settings.

In what circumstances could it be ethically defensible for a counsellor to report such information to someone with authority to act on it – the manager of an agency or principal of a school, for example – or to report the information directly to a statutory agency or to the police? As ordinary citizens we may have such concerns that the justification to act may seem morally compelling. As counsellors, our professional responsibilities and values, as well as ethical and legal guidelines, overlay everyday assumptions; priorities therefore become protecting the therapeutic relationship by observing the boundaries of confidentiality, while also working to prevent harm and "promote the safety and wellbeing" of others (NZAC *Code of Ethics*, 4.5).

If a client seeks a counsellor's support in passing information about illegal practices on to a third party such as a teacher, a statutory agency or the police, the request is unlikely to present an ethical dilemma. Before taking action, however, the reliability of the information and of its source needs to be considered. Within a school or a particular community, such information may be based on innuendo and rumour, and therefore more harm than good may eventuate if a counsellor takes action on this basis. If the information is hearsay, it would also be of limited value in the eyes of the police and the legal system.

However, when serious concern about illegal activities involving potential harm to the client or others is well-founded, a counsellor may consider taking action with or without the client's consent. Relevant clauses in the NZAC *Code of Ethics* that address matters of safety include 5.1a, the need to "take all reasonable steps to protect clients from harm", and 5.1d, a counsellor's duty to "warn third parties and appropriate authorities in the event of an imminent threat of serious harm to that third party from the client" (see Simon Jefferson, Part 4, section 1). Also pertinent are clauses delineating exceptions to confidentiality, particularly the first point under 6.2c, when "there is serious danger in the immediate or foreseeable future to the client or others."

A determination of what constitutes "an imminent threat" or "serious danger" cannot be speculative or retrospective, but must be grounded in a realistic assessment of the immediate circumstances, in the context in which they transpire. Counsellors are absolved from maintaining confidentiality only in specified circumstances, and "illegal practices" or "illegal activities" encompass a wide spectrum of possibilities, most of which would not be consistent with the Code's descriptions of an imminent threat of serious harm or serious danger.

Unlike ordinary citizens, or social workers who hold statutory powers, counsellors usually work from a paradigm in which they form private, fiduciary contracts with their clients that reflect the covenantal relationship between them (Ponton & Duba, 2009). The trust associated with this relationship is pivotal to the therapeutic effectiveness of any counselling process, and a higher level of "test" is therefore associated with a decision to convey information obtained in counselling to a third party. Counsellors working in cross-disciplinary teams or in more than one professional role within an agency may need to balance their responsibilities to NZAC with their accountability to agency policies and regulations. In any context, a major consideration is the question of the best course of action to safeguard the relationship between client and counsellor for the work of counselling, while at the same time addressing concerns regarding the wellbeing and safety of others who are affected by the illegal activities.

Concern about the devastating consequences of the manufacture and sale of methamphetamine or P, for example, may lead a counsellor to decide that this outweighs other factors, when hearing information from a client about a transaction that is about to take place. Such determinations are highly subjective, and consultation with a supervisor is essential as part of processes of ethical decision-making. Colin Hughes (see Part 3, Section 3) and Agee (1997) have discussed considerations that school counsellors are called upon to weigh up, when hearing information about drug-related or other illegal activities. In some situations, strategies can be developed that safeguard a therapeutic relationship while work is done with the help of third parties to intervene in such activities and minimise risk to others.

Counsellors working in community agencies and educational institutions can also play an important advocacy role in developing policies and protocols to guide staff in responding to information about illegal activities, in order to promote the safety of the community. In schools, for example, policies would concern matters such as drugs, violence and sexual abuse; in community agencies, policies regarding information about family violence would be a priority.

Hearing information about child abuse is one circumstance in which a counsellor's pathway forward is likely to be influenced by a variety of factors. These include:

- the circumstances in which the abuse is reported to be occurring;
- the age and vulnerability of the victim (who may or may not be the client);
- the current or imminent danger for the victim;
- the client's role in the scenario;
- the resources available to the client and to the victim; and
- the possible courses of action open to the client and to the counsellor.

Although reporting child abuse is not mandatory in New Zealand, under the Children, Young Persons and their Families Act 1989 anyone "who believes that a child under the age of 17 years has been, or is likely to be harmed (whether physically, emotionally, or sexually), ill-treated, abused, neglected, or deprived may report the matter to a departmental social worker or to a member of the police: s 15." If the report is made in good faith, the person making the report "is protected from any civil, criminal, or disciplinary proceedings: s 16" (Ludbrook, 2003, p. 177). To facilitate making fully informed decisions, counsellors need to be knowledgeable about reporting procedures as well as about the processes that are likely to ensue.

A challenging circumstance for a counsellor may occur when the desire to act on information about illegal practices cannot ethically be fulfilled, as is frequently the case. Counsellors may experience powerlessness and guilt about not being able to do anything to intervene, and the support of a supervisor and colleagues can be invaluable in addressing these reactions. Whatever pathway is appropriate in each unique situation, working with rather than against a client is likely to produce the most beneficial outcome for all concerned.

PART 5

WHEN THINGS GO WRONG

INTRODUCTION

Kathie Crocket

> We all make mistakes ... We all encounter risks in our everyday practice; thus [we] are vulnerable. Even the most careful and prudent practitioner ... (Shapiro, Walker, Manosevitz, Peterson & Williams, 2008, p. 3)

> Yes, mistakes, along with fecal matter, happen to us all. (Cummings, 2008, p. xix)

One aspect of maintaining competence is how we respond as counsellors when things go wrong. Part 1 introduced the idea of developing an ethical sensitivity that alerts us to the moment-by-moment ethical questions that arise in our practice, and from a relationally oriented, embodied ethics. But what about those moments that pass us by, when we do not notice an ethical question arising, but the moments are experienced by clients as unhelpful or worrying? Or those moments when we do notice but the moment passes without our giving consideration to what we noticed? Or moments that, at the time or later, appear to us clumsy or inept practice, but we do nothing in response for any number of reasons? Or when a client does not return and we have no sense whether or not the reason for that might be dissatisfaction with our practice? Or when client dissatisfaction is expressed through a formal complaint about a serious ethical concern? There are also those times when we may have counselled with ethical clarity, care and purpose, including through consultation in supervision, but a client or someone else sees things differently. Whether difficulties are identified by others, or by the counsellor, implications must be addressed. Practising within the scope of one's competence (NZAC *Code of Ethics*, 2002, 4.8), and upholding and fostering the values, integrity and ethics of the profession (8.2.a) is a counsellor's responsibility.

A profession's claims to autonomy are made on the basis of self-policed standards (Abbott & Wallace, 1990; Ramprogus, 1995). This policing or monitoring involves a range of strategies, at individual, local and professional level. On one hand, the desire to be in respectful relationship provides an altruistic kind of self-monitoring amongst individual counsellors, within supervisory dyads and local groups, and in the wider profession. And on the other hand, the social contract of a code of ethics and a complaints process produce a more disciplinary monitoring process, to which members of the profession agree to subject one another. In the first section that follows, Bob Manthei writes of the responsibilities counsellors have when a colleague's practice is impaired: the social contract we have as members of a profession means a position as uninvolved bystander is not available to us. A range of actions are possible – a formal complaint process is not likely to be the only potentially productive possibility. This is Sue Webb's point in the following section, when she reviews possible actions clients, and others, might take when something has, or appears to have, gone wrong in counselling. She makes the point that a complaints process will take a toll on all parties. In two sections of part 5, she offers guidance for complainants and respondents about managing themselves over the time of a complaints process. In the final section of part 5, Carol White outlines the Regional Ethics Process used by NZAC as one of the responses to complaints against its members.

5.1 WHEN A COLLEAGUE'S PRACTICE IS IMPAIRED

Bob Manthei

There are at least two categories of impairment to a counsellor's performance that can adversely affect their work with their colleagues, and more importantly, their clients:

- impairment due to personal, emotional or physical difficulties;
- impairment due to poor or erroneous judgement that results in unethical behaviour.

In both cases there is the risk that the counsellor may violate two of the NZAC's basic principles of ethical practice – avoiding doing harm in all their professional work, and practising within the scope of their competence – as well as the guideline of upholding and fostering the values, integrity and ethics of the profession. Apart from the potential for harming clients, both types of behaviour can also undermine the public's confidence in counselling. It is for these reasons that members have a responsibility, in a self-regulating professional counselling association such as NZAC, to take action when they become aware of another counsellor's impaired, incompetent or unethical behaviour. Counsellors have this responsibility to one another and to the counselling profession (7.1.a; 7.2.a; 7.3.a).

The dilemmas we may face when ethical concerns arise about a colleague's practice can be challenging and stressful, and the way forward may be far from clear-cut or easy. In practice, there are several things to consider carefully before acting, in order to ensure that the colleague about whom there is concern will be treated with respect, fairness and honesty *and* that clients are protected and receiving an acceptable level of counselling care (NZAC, 2002; Welfel, 2010).

The first category of impairment can include poor functioning due to illness (physical or mental), disability (such as hearing loss), drug use, personal or professional stress or distressing circumstances (such as depression, family circumstances or relationship difficulties, or problematic workplace policies), or even secondary post-traumatic stress for those working in crisis situations. Given the constant emotional demands on them, it is not surprising that some counsellors will experience these sorts of difficulties, or challenges that are associated with temporary or ongoing physical limitations. Counsellors themselves are responsible for maintaining their competence and monitoring their fitness to practice (5.9.a; 5.10), but there may also be times when they are unaware of their own limitations or cannot see their diminished performance clearly. This latter situation represents misconduct due to ignorance or erroneous interpretation of ethical principles and guidelines as outlined in a relevant code of ethics, and for members of NZAC this encompasses three types of behaviour (7.2.a):

- counsellor behaviour judged to be professional misconduct: "acting in contravention of the written and unwritten guidance of the profession" or service that has "fallen below the standards that would reasonably be expected of a practitioner exercising reasonable care and skill" (British Association for Counselling and Psychotherapy, 2010, p. 20);
- conduct unbecoming a member;
- conduct prejudicial to the interests of the Association: "the practitioner has acted in such an infamous or disgraceful way that the public's trust in the profession might be undermined" (British Association for Counselling and Psychotherapy, 2010, p. 20).

The first two types of behaviour are usually more straightforward than the third, mainly because they involve the way clients are being treated. These are areas that are discussed in some detail in the NZAC *Code of Ethics*. The third area, however, is more ambiguous and open to variable interpretations, particularly when it includes a colleague's relationship with other counsellors, colleagues or third parties, and individual beliefs about what constitutes effective counselling practice.

Although members of NZAC are expected to know and understand the *Code of Ethics* well enough to apply it in their work in a sensible and sensitive fashion, the code can only function as a guide and, accordingly, it is possible to misinterpret and misapply its principles. Thus, when counsellors learn of a colleague's unethical behaviour, they are required to consider that information carefully and thoroughly before deciding what action is most appropriate to take.

TAKING ACTION: A PROCESS OF CAREFUL ASSESSMENT AND CONSIDERED ACTION

When learning of a colleague's impaired counselling practice, counsellors have an ethical responsibility not to ignore it. In practice, this means carefully and systematically considering several important questions before deciding if a situation is serious enough to warrant taking further action:

- What is the nature and the seriousness of the reported impairment or ethical transgression? How frequent is the behaviour? How are people/clients affected by it? How many are affected?
- What is the source of your information and how accurate do you judge it to be? How trustworthy is the source? Where and how did they get the information, and how was it transmitted to you?
- If the source is a client report, what are the considerations with regard to client confidentiality, and a client's right to consent to any action that might be taken?
- What is your relationship with the counsellor who is the subject of the concern, or with the client, or other affected party? How does this relationship affect your reactions to this situation, your capacity to act, and possible courses of action?
- How injurious do you regard the behaviour to be, and to whom? What are the real and/or potential effects of the behaviour on clients, the community, the profession and NZAC?
- Which specific principles in the NZAC *Code of Ethics* are being violated and to what extent? How clear-cut, extensive or serious is the impairment or violation?
- Is there sufficient reason to think that the behaviour is serious enough to require further action?
- What options are open to you at this point, what are the benefits and risks associated with each, and which seems the most

sensible to follow? Is there a need to consult further, and with whom, before deciding upon a course of action? What is the best next step to take?

In thinking about these questions, it is a safeguard for everyone to consult with supervisors, or appropriate colleagues, in order to get additional perspectives on the situation. If there is urgency or a level of seriousness that poses a clear threat to a client's welfare, then a formal complaint or intervention should be initiated immediately, after discussion with a supervisor or trusted, experienced colleague.

If you decide that action is justified, it is normally recommended that you follow the simplest, quickest and least formal intervention possible to resolve the situation. Any action should involve treating a colleague with respect, fairness and honesty (7.1.a). The NZAC *Code of Ethics* sets out three possible actions that can be taken:

1. Discuss the situation with the counsellor concerned;
2. Notify the counsellor's supervisor, teacher or employer;
3. Use NZAC's formal complaints process.

In taking any action, the aim should be to work respectfully and cooperatively with the person who is the subject of the concern in order to maximise client care, and to preserve, protect and promote the reputation of both the profession and the association. There is no easy or clear guide for making decisions to act in this area of ethical practice. However, there are several steps, and things to consider at each step in the process, that may help clarify the implications of your obligations and how the situation can be dealt with in a constructive way.

Step 1: Accept and understand that the Code of Ethics guides counsellors towards taking action in response to apparently unethical or incompetent behaviour by colleagues (7.2). This step requires an understanding of what a self-regulating profession is, what it stands for, how it works, and what members' responsibilities include. It also means accepting the uncertainty of not knowing if one's interpretation of another's behaviour is 'correct'; having the confidence to deal with the matter in a direct, honest and constructive way at all times; having the courage to risk incurring the hostility of a colleague; and having the commitment and conviction to see the process through to its conclusion.

Step 2: Develop an understanding of how to assess the seriousness of the behaviour in question. In order to take action on a concern about a colleague's behaviour, it must first be shown to be a sufficiently 'serious' ethical breach to warrant further intervention. It is not sufficient to target behaviour that is merely based on a difference in philosophy, personality, cultural practice, religious belief or sexual orientation, or to act in a way that is based on discrimination, personal jealousy, affront or insult. Violation of any of the nine ethical principles listed in the NZAC *Code of Ethics* (4.1–4.9) would constitute questionable and serious behaviour.

Step 3: Once there is sufficient evidence that there has been behaviour serious enough to take further action, how does one proceed? In most cases the recommended first step is to discuss the matter with the colleague personally, outside the bounds of any formal complaints procedure (Corey, Corey & Callanan, 2007) This is important for reasons of fairness and respectfulness. It may be the case that the colleague has a different and perfectly acceptable explanation or rationale for their behaviour. If an informal approach is not successful, then a more formal pathway can be followed, such as raising the matter with the colleague's supervisor, employer, private practice partner, or, ultimately, by lodging a formal complaint. Once a colleague's behaviour has been identified formally, the matter must be taken seriously and investigated according to published processes.

If the colleague is a member of a different professional association, or not a member of any association, it may still be possible to talk informally with them – clearly, honestly, dispassionately – about the behaviour, and suggest that they review their practice, preferably in their supervision sessions. If the identity of a supervisor is known, and the behaviour is reported to a supervisor, the supervisor then has a duty to discuss it with the counsellor. This action can be a useful and relatively low-key way of ensuring that a counsellor's questionable behaviour is reviewed.

Step 4: Be prepared to remain involved in some capacity until the matter is fully resolved. Once a counsellor takes some action, informal or formal, about a colleague's behaviour, there is an obligation to participate until the matter is finally settled. This participation may include being asked to discuss the impaired behaviour with the counsellor, giving evidence formally or informally, and supporting one's reasoning orally or in writing. For a counsellor's own legal protection and in fairness to the person about whom the complaint is made, it is important to be well researched, clear and factual. There is likely to be personal stress involved, since it is not easy to confront colleagues about inappropriate or unethical behaviour, and there may be some degree of retaliation and criticism from the person who is the subject of the complaint and/or from other practitioners (Clarkson, 2001). On the other hand, colleagues may admire the courage and professionalism shown, and some will be grateful that the counsellor taking action chose not to be a bystander and ignore the situation, but chose to act responsibly and ethically (Clarkson, 2001).

5.2
TO COMPLAIN OR NOT TO COMPLAIN: THAT IS THE QUESTION

Sue Webb

There can be a number of reasons for things not going well in counselling and a number of possible responses, one of which is to lodge a formal complaint. This section looks at approaches to addressing difficulties in counselling. It considers whether to lodge a formal complaint from three perspectives: that of clients, clients' friends or family members, and finally, from fellow counsellors. It is important that clients and those connected to them find avenues to express and address concerns, whether or not these turn out to relate to unethical behaviour on the part of counsellors.

TO COMPLAIN OR NOT: FOR CLIENTS

Knowing whether counselling is progressing as it should is not always straightforward. Exploring personal difficulties and making changes are often not easy tasks and sometimes problems which are familiar can seem to provide a sort of comfort, making change quite disorienting. Feeling upset when leaving the counselling room and spending time afterwards going over what has been discussed can be signs that counselling is working well. Some approaches also suggest that, at times, clients can develop quite negative feelings towards their counsellors, termed "negative transference" (Corey, 2009), especially if working on earlier relationships in which these feelings were not experienced fully at the time or were not allowed expression. According to these approaches, it is therapeutic for a client to experience and express negative feelings towards a counsellor in a safe and constructive way.

However, a sense of ongoing dissatisfaction with an aspect of counselling, or with the overall progress of counselling, deserves attention. There are two ways in which a client's[1] counselling may be problematic: the counsellor may be acting inappropriately, for example by insisting the client undertake certain behaviours, by breaking confidentiality, or by attending to other matters during the appointment time. Alternatively, there may be things that a practitioner is failing to do, such as not referring the client to another service when the counsellor is unable to help further, or not addressing the real issues of concern, so that nothing is changing for the client. The first sort of unethical behaviour is perhaps noticed more readily than the second. It may be helpful to read through the NZAC *Code of Ethics* (2002) and/or the Health and Disability Code (Health and Disability Commissioner, 2004), to consult a book (for example, Manthei & Miller, 2000), to talk through concerns with someone else – preferably with some experience of counselling themselves – or to try writing about the experiences.

Once the dissatisfaction is clarified, and if it seems possible that the situation could be improved, raising the concern with the counsellor is an important option to consider. Alternatively, other possibilities may be to end the counselling, without taking any further action, or to change counsellors. However, when a counsellor has behaved harmfully or dangerously, a formal complaint is appropriate. It may take some courage, time and careful thought to decide to do this, including weighing up the personal resources a complaint may require.

Should the client want to continue the counselling, difficulties might be addressed through discussion or by sending the counsellor a letter or email. It is possible to request a separate meeting, without incurring a charge, to discuss the concerns, perhaps taking along a support person. Before doing this, it is important to clarify what outcome is desired, such as an apology and/or a change in how the work is undertaken. The counsellor could also be asked to take the issue to supervision. If writing, it is worth consulting with someone supportive about how best to express the difficulties. How the counsellor handles the issues raised will provide information that can be helpful in deciding what to do next.

1 Through these sections I have tended to use the singulars 'client', 'friend' etc, rather than 'client or clients', 'friend or friends' etc in the interests of brevity. The sections also refer, however, to counselling that may take place with more than one client at a time, who may together experience dissatisfaction. Similarly friends, family members or counsellors may wish to take action together to challenge inappropriate counselling.

If the response does not prove helpful, the way forward may be to end the counselling.

Ending the counselling may be sufficient. It may, however, be that the counsellor's response continues to cause concern, or indicates that others may also be at risk. If appropriate, and if the client wants to take the matter to a further level, the counsellor's manager – if they have one – and/or their supervisor could be approached and told of the difficulties. This might be done face-to-face, perhaps with a support person, or in writing, with some careful preparation as to what the implications might be for the client – for example, in relation to privacy – and how best to present the issues.

The final option is to lodge a formal complaint with the professional association, an employer, or the Health and Disability Commissioner (HDC). The latter would be the obvious choice if the matter seemed too serious to be addressed less formally, or other approaches had not proved satisfactory. Further information on formal complaints to NZAC can be obtained from the NZAC website, under "Ethics" http://www.nzac.org.nz, or by emailing the Ethics Secretary, ethicssecretary@nzac.org.nz. NZAC, as well as giving written information, can provide a procedural adviser to help explain the complaints process.

TO COMPLAIN OR NOT: FOR RELATIVES AND FRIENDS

Sometimes close friends or relatives of clients have a sense that counselling is not happening appropriately. This can be particularly difficult, because for the most part third parties do not have direct evidence of the counselling. It is less complex for third parties to address a problem if the client agrees with their perspectives. It is important for relatives or friends to discuss with the client whether they would be interested in taking some sort of action, either with or without support. Considering the problem in relation to the NZAC and HDC codes named above may help to focus the discussion.

However, the client may not see things in the same way as someone close to them. They may perhaps have become dependent on the counsellor; or they may perceive their relationship with the family member or friend to be part of the difficulties they are addressing in counselling. Unless the concerned person has independent evidence – for example, of interactions observed between the client and counsellor, or evidence of financial deceit or of emotional deterioration that can be connected directly to counselling sessions – attempts to intervene in or complain about the client's counselling are likely to be difficult. Taking the power out of the client's hands may make things worse for that person, and may damage the third party's own relationship with them in the process. It may be best to be patient and wait to see if the client in time comes to agree that the counselling is problematic.

It is important for others in a client's life to recognise that their own relationship with the client may temporarily be more fraught while changes develop as a result of the counselling. Change in a familiar other can be difficult to adjust to. It might be helpful to consider to what extent they would see the changes as problematic, were they not close to this person and familiar with their past behaviour. The client may also at times react inappropriately to dynamics that have hurt them in other relationships. This can be a particular problem for parents and partners. Patience may determine whether the difficulties pass in time.

However, situations can occur in which a third party might take considered action, without the approval of a client. This could include when the client appears in grave danger, seemingly as a result of the counselling. For example, the client could be becoming increasingly depressed, suicidal, self-destructive or physically abusive of others.

If a third party chooses to approach the counsellor about the concerns, it is important to be aware that the counsellor cannot disclose anything about either the client or the counselling, without the client's permission. If the client is a child, elderly person or person with an intellectual disability, what can be shared with others directly concerned in the client's care is something the counsellor should clarify at the outset and routinely check at the end of each counselling session. Confidentiality is at the core of responsible counselling. A concerned person, however, is not bound by any formal code to maintain confidentiality. They might provide a counsellor with information that could be helpful in working with the client. A limited or guarded response to a third party's disclosure does not mean that the counsellor has not taken account of what has been conveyed.

Third parties can be concerned that a counsellor may be encouraging a client to believe lies about them, which are contributing to deterioration in their relationship with the client. It is often the case that others are unduly worried about the extent to which they are the focus of the counselling. It can also happen that clients may say something like, "My counsellor says ..." to try to add weight to their own position in a disagreement. Effective counselling does not involve the counsellor delivering judgements on clients or others. Should concerns about counselling content lead to a desire to access the counsellor's notes, according to the Privacy Act 1993, only those parts that clearly relate to a particular person can be made available to that person. For the most part, counsellors do not specifically identify people other than the client in their notes.

There have been instances, in New Zealand and elsewhere, in which a client's relative or partner has taken their hurt and anger about counselling to the press. Unfortunately, media involvement can easily go awry and the person risks becoming caught up in self-exposure and self-justification they had not foreseen. In addition, it may subject the client to unwanted media attention and further damage the relationship between the client and the relative through the public airing of interpersonal difficulties.

An alternative step, if a counsellor has already been approached or the counselling appears harmful, may be to contact the counsellor's employer, if they have one. Many organisations have systems for managing complaints and concerns about their employees. The employer may also be able to provide advice as to where else the difficulty might be taken; for example, to the counsellor's supervisor.

Finally, a complaint can be lodged with a counsellor's professional association or with the Health and Disability Commissioner, if there is sufficient direct evidence for this to be investigated. This will be easier if the client supports the action and may be prepared to give permission, for example, for others to access their notes. Hearsay information (that is, a third party's account of what others, including the client, may have recounted but are not prepared to complain about directly themselves) is unlikely to be sufficient on its own to result in a complaint being upheld, unless the counsellor admits to the behaviour complained about.

TO COMPLAIN OR NOT: FOR COUNSELLORS

The NZAC *Code of Ethics* (2002) recommends to counsellors that they treat colleagues with respect, fairness and honesty (7.1.a), and take action when they consider another counsellor's behaviour could be judged unethical (7.2.a). The *Code of Ethics* suggests three levels of action: addressing the matter with the counsellor; notifying their supervisor, teacher or employer; or using the formal complaints process. The decision as to what to do will be determined by both the seriousness of the alleged behaviour and the evidence the colleague has.

Examples of directly observed behaviour might include: disrespectful conduct by a colleague during karakia, which could be addressed directly with the counsellor; a practitioner overstepping the limits of their competence several times, which might lead a supervisor to approach the employer; or a counsellor defending an intimate relationship with a recent client because their supervisor had approved it, which would most likely merit a formal complaint. Less easy are situations such as: an individual client reporting a lack of even-handedness in their couples counselling through the Family Court; talk amongst NZAC branch members about the apparent increasing memory difficulties of a senior branch member; or the reported approval by a supervisor of the intimate relationship cited above. Many concerns are likely, at least initially, to benefit from a more informal approach.

Raising concerns with a colleague, whether formally or informally, should be understood as an act of kindness and courage; doing so may help a counsellor return to ethical practice and can prevent more serious or more widespread lapses later. Taking action does, however, require good self-management. A guiding principle might be that we act towards our colleagues as we would hope they would act towards us, were our roles reversed – an application of the ancient 'Golden Rule' common to many religions – while also taking into account the point that compassion alone is it is not sufficient to ensure ethical practice (Hugman, 2005).

As with concerns about the counselling involving a family member or friend, colleagues require direct evidence of alleged inappropriate behaviour, not merely reports from third parties, if a formal complaint is to be lodged. However, less certain evidence does not prevent an informal approach to the counsellor, the counsellor and supervisor, and/or the counsellor and their manager, drawing on reliable sources. Furthermore, consistent reports of concerning behaviour from different sources would suggest some value in following these up in some way. If three separate clients, for example, talked of dismissive behaviour by the same counsellor, this would suggest a difficulty needing attention.

In approaching the problem informally, it is necessary to protect the safety and interests of those who have supplied the information, especially if they are former clients of the counsellor. Taking action is more readily mandated when those concerned ask for or agree to action being taken. In giving permission, clients have a right to hear a full account of what will be addressed, and how. If permission has not been given, proceeding may be very difficult because clients' identities must be protected and therefore concerns may only be able to be expressed in a general way. So, for example, a counsellor might be restricted to pointing out that there were reports of disrespectful behaviour, because informing the colleague that an ex-client had complained of swearing and shouting in sessions might lead to the counsellor identifying the person concerned. In such cases it may be preferable to patiently support the ex-client in ways that may ultimately enable them to act on their own behalf, or to give others permission to do so.

Beyond the collegial, informal approach, it may be necessary – either because the behaviour is of serious concern or if other avenues have failed – to consider more formal action. The more formal the intended action, the more necessary it will be to have first-hand evidence of the behaviour at issue. A more formalised approach may be made to the supervisor or employer, or a formal complaint made to the counsellor's professional association or the HDC. Professional respect for the counsellor would recommend telling them of the concerns and the actions taken, unless this might put either valuable evidence or other people at risk.

Being involved in a complaint against a colleague, either formal or informal, is not easy. It may involve difficult interaction with someone who is likely to be part of the counsellor's own professional community, potentially resulting in other, more everyday relations becoming strained, at least for a while. There may be multiple relationships among the counsellors, supervisors and/or employers who participate in addressing the concern. Affective responses will be likely to influence participants' perceptions, particularly in situations of apparently serious breaches of the NZAC *Code of Ethics*; it is our responsibility to attend to our own competence, including experiences of shame, fear, dismay and disgust, during our participation in any actions involving our colleagues.

CONCLUSION

Deciding to complain or not, whether as a client, family member, friend or colleague, is never straightforward. It involves weighing up not only the rights and wrongs of the situation as perceived by the potential complainant, but also the nature of the evidence available, the processes that may be involved, and the likely emotional resources needed to undertake the complaint. These, in turn, may determine whether it is appropriate to begin with an informal or a formal approach. The next two sections will consider the experience of the formal complaints process from the complainant's and the respondent's perspectives.

5.3 ON BEING A COMPLAINANT

Sue Webb

This section offers assistance for those who have decided to lodge a complaint. It describes aspects of complaints processes, focusing on those of the NZAC, while considering some common difficulties that complainants may experience and offering some strategies that may help.

COMPLAINTS PROCESSES

It is important to understand the purpose of a complaints process in order to hold realistic expectations as to its outcome. Its main aim is neither to punish a respondent nor to heal a complainant's hurt, but to educate and create greater safety for clients, both in relation to an individual counsellor and within the profession in general. Once a concern is formally expressed and accepted, the complaint is no longer merely a matter between a client and a counsellor; "ownership" for determining questions about the ethics of practice and responsibility for upholding these are placed with the body to which the complaint has been made. While sometimes this shift can appear to "sideline" a complainant, the process enacts the profession's responsibility to its community.

A clear sense of purpose can be important in sustaining the decision to complain. Formal complaints processes are rarely quick, and energy may need to be sustained over a longer period than might be imagined. Support from family, friends and, if relevant and acceptable, another counsellor, can make the process less burdensome, distressing or lonely. As with matters taken to court, it is important to recognise that there is no guarantee that the complainant's desired outcome will result, even when a complaint is justified. It may be helpful to consider how to cope with potentially unwanted outcomes, as well as possible delays. Sometimes making a complaint brings an immediate sense of relief or satisfaction; at other times the process can seem counterproductive.

SUBMITTING A COMPLAINT TO A HEARING BODY

A written account of what happened needs to be submitted, telling the story as clearly as possible, in the order in which events happened. Maintaining a perspective on what was problematic and what was not can be useful. While consideration of the relevant clauses of the appropriate code of ethics may be helpful, there is no obligation to do this, since it is the job of the profession's ethics representatives to identify the specific clauses that are relevant and which matters of concern are within its scope.

Once the account is written, it may seem embarrassing or uncomfortable to share it. If the person complaining is unsure about carrying through with the complaint, it is perfectly possible to delay, providing this does not take a number of years. Some people find sharing something that has been secret, and that perhaps has also felt shameful, makes them feel stronger. However, it is possible to withdraw or suspend a complaint once it is underway, if continuing is too difficult. As each new stage of the process is reached, there is usually time to prepare emotionally for what is to come.

WHILE THE COMPLAINT IS UNDERWAY

NZAC provides full information about its complaints process, both on its website (www.nzac.org.nz) and through the Ethics Secretary, who will also offer to refer a complainant to an NZAC procedural adviser. The advisors are available to help the complainant understand the process, explain written information sent or clarify steps along the way. If there is no one else to call on, they can also help the complainant to work out how to express the complaint in writing, or act as support person at a hearing. If there are questions they cannot answer, they can be asked to contact the ethics secretary, or the complainant can do this themselves.

Once a complaint has been accepted as potentially serious enough to warrant further investigation, a complainant becomes a witness in the case NZAC takes to investigate the complaint, either by a hearing for potentially serious ethical breaches, or through the use of a regional ethics team, employing a more informal and educative approach. Either way, the complainant's role is to provide the information that enables the NZAC ethics team to take the matter up with the counsellor.

Communications from the NZAC Ethics Secretary are usually quite brief, using a neutral tone and providing only limited information. This is because the process a complaints body undertakes must be fair, impartial and legally defensible. For a complaint to be upheld or sanctions imposed on a counsellor, a process that follows the rules of "natural justice" (Binmore, 2005) must be used. "Natural justice" broadly means the enactment of fair play.

Laying a complaint can be stressful and it can be difficult to keep a sense of proportion. For example, it is possible to become over-anxious about the hurt the counsellor may experience; or conversely, a sense of injustice about the concerns may persuade the complainant that the counsellor is a much worse person than is reasonable. Complainants, who have often lost a sense of trust in and control over their counselling, may struggle to relinquish control to the professional body and to trust in its procedures. Nonetheless, the responsibility for the decision-making rests squarely with the professional body once a complaint has been made.

The complaints process takes considerable time, and patience may be required. The timeframe is again due to the need for natural justice; both the complainant and the respondent counsellor are given time to consult others and formulate responses. In addition, the association draws on voluntary assistance from its members to examine complaints. This work needs to fit alongside their other responsibilities, and occasionally their lives can be subject to sudden change and crisis. In addition, small teams of members work on complaints, and decision-making by a group tends to take time.

AFTERWARDS

Once the complaints process is finished, complainants may find themselves feeling lighter and able to move on. However, some may experience the outcome as less than they had hoped for. Complainants also at times feel dissatisfied at not having actually witnessed justice taking place, since many complaints processes, including NZAC's, do not have the complainant present throughout the process and do not make detailed information on the findings available afterwards. This does not mean that the counsellor was not properly called to account. Whatever the outcome, it is important to bear in mind that the complaint will have led the counsellor to examine their practice in great detail, to discuss it thoroughly with their supervisor, and to explain themselves to colleagues. It is rare for some sort of educational benefit not to emerge from this process. While the complainant may also feel inclined to want some responsibility for ensuring any sanctions are correctly carried out, this is the complaints body's task.

Making and seeing through a complaint is likely to be a challenging experience for complainants. However, without the effort made by complainants, counselling associations would not be able to monitor individual members and assist them to function more appropriately and skilfully, or to identify when membership of a professional association should be downgraded or withdrawn. Trends in complaints also serve to inform a professional body such as NZAC about areas of risk that can then become the subject of educational and training activities. In the long term, complainants may discover that they too have gained from the process, in ways that may not have been obvious at the time.

5.4 ON BEING A RESPONDENT

Sue Webb

In any professional career, there may be occasions when practice in some way falls short of agreed professional ethical standards, even in the presence of careful self and professional monitoring. This section considers how counsellors might respond when a momentary lapse, an unconsidered absence of care, or a more serious transgression has effects that lead to a complaint being made about their practice. Complaints might be made to practitioners directly, to counsellors' employers, to the professional association, or to the Health and Disability Commissioner. Whatever the circumstances, a code of ethics plays a core role in guiding practitioners' responses.

Whether a complaint is voiced directly by a client, conveyed indirectly by a colleague or other third party to whom the client has spoken, or received by means of a formal letter from a professional body, it can come as a surprise and a shock. Acknowledging and addressing strong feelings are an integral part of our professional responsibilities as counsellors (see Bill Grant, Part 3, Section 10), becoming particularly important in managing the complicated responses a complaint may evoke. While we have the responsibility and right to care appropriately for ourselves, it is also our duty to think in terms of care for the complainant: a complaint does not absolve us of our professional responsibilities towards a client.

For example, a client discloses her disappointment that in a previous counselling session she felt more attention had been paid to her children than to her own struggles and needs. The surprise and distress that a counsellor might experience on hearing this can be processed later in supervision. In the moment, the client's needs must take priority, including understanding and clarifying more about what, in particular, she experienced as unhelpful or unethical. It could also be helpful to offer her the option of writing about her concern. This writing could also be valuable in addressing the matter in supervision. If it becomes clear what caused the difficulty, a potential rupture in the relationship may be resolved immediately if the counsellor apologises, and if mutual understanding is re-established. Another possible outcome, however, may be an agreement to end the counselling relationship. The models provided by Welfel (2005, 2010) – acknowledging the violation, assessing and responding to the damage caused, and rehabilitating the counsellor – offer valuable frameworks for addressing one's own mistakes. Managing these processes with grace brings together the professional and the personal.

Where a complaint first emerges in a more formal, public domain, such as at work or via the professional association, both our own affective responses and our formal responses are likely to be more complex. This section focuses on responding in these more formal situations, using some of NZAC's processes as the context in which to discuss personal and professional self-care and self-management through a complaints process. Less official complaints or those handled informally within the workplace, while probably less stressful, will also engender some of the same responses, and require similar strategies.

THE INITIAL REACTION

The receipt of a complaint is potentially traumatic. An anonymous British counsellor ('Chris', 2001) provided a vivid account of the shame, fear, anger, and sense of betrayal and persecution experienced. However, it is important to stay realistic about the extent of the risk to professional life. While something inappropriate may have taken place, only a small number of counsellors will have breached the *Code of Ethics* in ways that suggest they should no longer be in practice (Winslade & White, 2002). Most commonly, complaints evoke a period of sustained self-examination, and sanctions may include an apology, additional education, targeted supervisory help, and perhaps temporarily ceasing work with a particular group of clients. Occasionally, membership status may be downgraded, but this is rare. Accounts of complaints procedures internationally (for example, Strom-Gottfried, 2003) mirror the frequency of corrective action, as opposed to more serious outcomes.

A complaint may be not at all, partly, or completely justified. Whatever the case, a complainant's concern needs to be addressed, and a fair process undertaken to examine it. Flight, fight or freeze will not be helpful responses (Paton, 2003). Clear thinking and action can be hindered if one becomes distracted by a sense of injustice; if one assumes that others will immediately see a complaint as unreasonable; or, conversely, if one engages in generalised self-recrimination. A wise respondent considers carefully what actually took place, how best to respond, how to find support, and how to manage other aspects of life, through what can at times seem a drawn-out and painful process.

A complaint, however, tends to strike not just at the professional self, but at the personal too. The person of the counsellor is central to the working relationship, so any failure in a counselling relationship is likely to be experienced as an attack on self-concept generally. It may be helpful therefore to remember that the complaint is about a specific piece of work, not the entirety of either a counsellor's professional activities or personhood.

It is also professionally important to separate the complaint from the person complaining. Sometimes those who lodge complaints may have been difficult to work with and/or have had complex needs, and there can be a temptation to blame a complainant, or cast doubts on their state of mind. The responsibility for maintaining a safe and effective working relationship, however, belongs with the counsellor. At the very least, the complainant and the counsellor have experienced rupture regarding the matter complained of. It is important, therefore, that a counsellor takes time to consider calmly whether there might have been an ethical breach, small or large, and how that might have occurred.

Similarly, blaming the investigating person or body, or finding fault with the processes instigated, may distract from the real task at hand. It is an employer's or a professional association's task to guard the reputation and interests of the organisation, or of counselling in general; to promote safe functioning; and to furnish good feedback to those investigated. It is also their responsibility to attempt to satisfy any complainant's concerns. Responses should not be in blind defence of an employee or a member of an association.

FOCUSING ON THE SELF

A number of counsellors' difficulties are associated with overlooking and neglecting to address personal issues (Schoener, Milgrom, Gonsiorek, Leupker & Conroe, 1989; Welfel, 2010). A range of situations can lead to enacting in some way, with clients or colleagues, matters that require personal and professional attention: overwork; inappropriately invested needs in client relationships; disenchantment with working and/or personal life; depression; poor organisation; an unrealistic view of competencies; problematic feelings; family worries; isolation; and/or poor self-concept. Ideally, these common difficulties are identified and dealt with in the course of supervision, or, if necessary, through seeking help elsewhere. Faced with a complaint, it may be helpful to look beyond the complaint itself to what, in a more general way, might have fuelled the difficulty from within the counsellor's personal and/or professional life. Even if personal difficulties did not underlie the circumstances of the complaint, such self-reflection can assist a counsellor in working through the emotional effects of a complaint and avoiding the development of attendant difficulties.

WHO TO INCLUDE

Who should know about a complaint, what help can be accessed, and how much can be discussed? Whether or not there is a contracted requirement, it is advisable to notify one's supervisor, an employer, funding agency and/or any insurer as soon as possible. At a personal level, those closest to the respondent may best be able to provide effective support in dealing with the shame and other painful emotions that a complaint may evoke, and in putting matters in perspective. It is also possible that, at some stage, a respondent might want to seek counselling.

It is important, however, to think carefully about how widely information should spread and where to expect support (Jamieson, 2001). The respondent is bound by confidentiality not to share information about the complainant outside supervision or counselling. This limitation may include details of the complaint itself, but it does not prevent a counsellor from talking about their own process and feelings: shame and isolation are unhelpful. Good supporters are those who can listen, respond to feelings, not pass judgement on either respondent or complainant, and remain grounded as to the overall impact of this event on the respondent's identity. Joining the respondent in blaming the complainant and/or the complaints process will not help to keep matters in perspective or facilitate courageous self-examination, if that is necessary.

Seeking support indiscriminately from professional colleagues may prove unhelpful. Some may have difficulty being honest in responding, especially if they believe that an ethical breach may have occurred. For most counsellors, the potential for being in receipt of a complaint can generate quite intense feelings, especially fear, which may skew their responses or, alternatively, lead to a distancing from the respondent (Thomas, 2005). There is also the risk that local professional communities can split into camps for and against the complaint, with colleagues finding it hard to hold a not-knowing position amidst the tensions generated.

Taking legal advice can be valuable at the outset, particularly if facing a formal hearing process and if the outcomes might affect employment or earning power. However, the expense and effort may not be merited if a lesser outcome is likely. Lawyers understand the culture of the law, which may be unfamiliar to most counsellors, and can provide clear information that can offer reassurance. Their training is to focus logically and dispassionately on the content and procedures at hand, and to evaluate potential courses of action. However, there have been occasions when the adversarial stance of a legal culture has been at odds with a more restorative counselling culture. For example, tactics such as unnecessary delaying may undermine goodwill. The habits of court performance may sit uncomfortably within the less formal context of a counselling ethics complaints hearing. If a lawyer is engaged, these factors can be weighed and discussed at the outset, and monitored throughout.

PROFESSIONAL SELF-CARE

Professional self-care will involve both reviewing what may have gone awry in the counselling, and taking account of the impact of the complaint itself. Is the self in equilibrium (Dunnett, 2009)? Should the caseload be reduced, or work with some types of client suspended, or more attention paid to non-work matters? Should more frequent supervision be engaged in, or personal counselling undertaken, or burnout addressed? Normal clear-sightedness and judgement may be compromised, so paying attention to the views of a trusted supervisor or colleague can be invaluable.

Fear and powerlessness can lead to a desire to direct and control. However, attempts to influence the outcome of the process by assuming inappropriate roles or taking unconsidered action may create further risk. How a counsellor handles a complaint can be at least as significant as the substance of the complaint. Also, staying within the boundaries of the allotted role of "respondent to a complaint", and focusing on undertaking this role to the best of one's ability, can contribute to a well-functioning process, and to reaching a fair outcome.

ACCESSING PROFESSIONAL HELP

Good supervision can be central to responding effectively to a complaint, whether or not the issue concerned has previously been discussed there. A supervisor, however, may need to manage both their own insecurity in the face of the complaint, and their fears of being found wanting as a supervisor. Becoming part of a poorly functioning dynamic is not useful (Dunnett, 2009), so a supervisor's own supervision may assist in avoiding unhelpful self-blame, counsellor blame, or premature rejection of a complainant's perspective.

The supervisory process can deepen understanding of what has happened, and provide opportunities to experiment with alternative perspectives, and theorise these constructively. It can also offer exploration of links between the personal and the professional, and challenge any blind spots. In enabling the respondent to stay connected to the reality of the situation, supervision can facilitate the development of wise responding strategies. By contrast, a supervisor who blindly champions the counsellor, becomes outraged at the complaint, or expresses distrust of organisational processes is unhelpful.

Central to effective supervision is a supervisor's capacity to examine, challenge and confront in ways that accept and support a respondent, facilitating valuable professional learning while accompanying them through the complaints process. The supervisor has responsibility to the respondent and the profession. Where supervision does not cover these dimensions, it may be important to seek additional, or alternative, supervisory support.

The NZAC complaints processes have provision for a respondent to use a procedural advisor selected from a list. This person can talk through various options, explain the processes, and act as a conduit for information from the ethics secretary, should the respondent feel unable to seek this for themselves. The advisor's task is not to side with a respondent but to facilitate their understanding of, and progression through, the complaints process.

Counselling may also be helpful as a source of support within a highly stressful situation to assist a respondent with self-examination, as well as to provide a safe context in which to address one's own and others' reactions, and to explore different responses. It can offer the respondent both the luxury of attending solely to the self, and freedom to be emotionally honest and personally vulnerable in a confidential context.

GAINING PERSPECTIVE

Amidst whatever turmoil the complaint causes, it can be important to establish some cognitive anchors to develop understanding and provide additional perspectives. This might occur alone, in supervision, through counselling, or with relevant peers, and might employ a range of conceptual frameworks. Library research and reading may facilitate the development of a deeper and more detailed position on what has taken place. That, in turn, may assist the counsellor to articulate more profound and considered responses to the complaint. Theoretical understandings might then be extended to identify potential strategies for repairing any damage that may have occurred – to either respondent or complainant.

ATTENDING TO THE NON-COUNSELLING SELF

Central to managing the process of responding to a complaint is attending to the non-counselling self. Being complained about can feel overwhelming and absorbing, making it easy to forget that there are other aspects to being. The maintenance and care of one's everyday self can help sustain both the emotional resilience and the cognitive attention necessary (Thomas, 2005).

It may be timely to set about re-examining one's identity, values and hopes. An audit of the physical, emotional, cognitive, social and spiritual aspects of self may reveal that activities and involvements previously precious, and part of a general sense of well-being, have reduced or disappeared. It may help to renew engagement in activities and experiences outside of professional life, to provide an alternative focus, and to support well-being.

RESPONDING ETHICALLY TO THE COMPLAINT

Finally, a respondent, in collaboration with their supervisor, needs to set about developing a response to the complaint, using a systematic, in-depth and good-willed approach. Working carefully through the complaint, identifying and attempting to respond in a reasoned way to each key ethical issue raised, will address the complaint thoroughly, and may reduce the need for further requests for information. Counselling notes, reports, diary entries, and supervision notes – respondent's and supervisor's – may be relevant.

In the process of working through the complaint material, it may become clear to a respondent that some errors were made, whether these were ones identified in the complaint or not. If so, these can be discussed fully in supervision, and acknowledged in the written response. If relevant, steps can be taken to remove the risk of recurrence, including possibly ceasing work with a particular client group until better equipped to do so. Since complaints processes have a tendency to take longer than all parties would like, a respondent may find it helpful to initiate remedial action themselves; for example, relevant professional development, targeted supervision, consultation or personal counselling. These initiatives should only occur, however, after consulting sufficiently to be clear about what may be helpful. A respondent should resist any temptation to involve the complainant.

THE OUTCOME

The best outcome for a respondent is to have participated respectfully in a complaints process that was constructive in providing education, facilitating safety, offering usable feedback, and stimulating change, if these were found to be necessary. The benefits may only emerge, however, with some distance from the experience itself. Valuable learning may derive from painful experiences and may lead in unforeseen directions. To conduct oneself with dignity, commitment and integrity requires a resilient, honest and constantly attentive relationship with oneself, both professionally and personally.

5.5
THE NZAC REGIONAL ETHICS PROCESS

Carol White

Over time, NZAC has developed complaints processes to accompany the *Code of Ethics* (2002). If a client believes that a counsellor has behaved in unethical ways, the client may complain to the association, which has a national ethics committee, charged with responding to expressions of concern or complaint. Currently, all but the most serious complaints are dealt with at regional level, through the work of regional ethics teams (RET).

RESPONDING TO COMPLAINTS

All concerns or complaints to NZAC must relate to a named member or provisional member. Complaints must be submitted in writing to the Ethics Secretary. The first step in the process is to determine whether the behaviour complained about is potentially prejudicial to the interests of NZAC, or potentially constitutes professional misconduct or conduct unbecoming a member. If a concern meets these criteria, NZAC will send a letter to the complainant outlining the association's complaints process. If consent is granted by the complainant, their letter of concern is then forwarded to the counsellor (who becomes known as the respondent). Once the respondent has provided the ethics secretary with a response to the concern, the Initial Assessment Group (IAG) – made up of the Ethics Convenor, the Ethics Secretary and one member from the National Ethics Committee – carefully considers which of four possible courses of action to follow, and the Ethics Secretary informs the respondent of the decision. The possible courses of action are to:

- provide assistance to the complainant to seek private resolution;
- take no further action;
- refer the complaint to the local RET;
- proceed to a formal hearing (conducted by members of the national ethics committee).

The focus of this section is the third of these courses of action, the regional process.

The association has regional ethics teams throughout the country. Members are nominated by branches, and their membership confirmed by the national executive. Each team is led by a member of NZAC's National Ethics Committee.

THE REGIONAL ETHICS PROCESS (REP)

This process applies to complaints about counsellor behaviour which is assessed as potentially at a mild or moderate level of seriousness. Appropriate cultural processes are implemented, if either or both the complainant and/or respondent are Māori.

INTENTIONS OF THE REP

The process is designed to provide both parties – the complainant and the respondent – with the opportunity to each speak directly and privately with RET members. It is a unique pathway, neither hearing nor mediation, and educative rather than disciplinary. The REP has been designed to enable NZAC to:

- formulate an understanding of the circumstances that led to the complaint being made;
- identify any ways in which the respondent may have contributed to the situation, and if this is found to be the case;
- propose restorative and/or educative actions to minimise the likelihood of such events recurring.

Where it is identified that there has been behaviour prejudicial to the interests of NZAC, or that constitutes professional misconduct or conduct unbecoming a member, the REP offers opportunity for a respondent to acknowledge mistakes made and to act to improve their practice. When a complaint is addressed through the REP the matter is closed when the

RET members are satisfied with the outcome. If they are not satisfied, the complaint may be referred back to the convenor of the ethics committee.

The RET members carefully investigate the complaint and the process is potentially restorative.

PROCEDURAL ADVISORS

All RET members are available to act as procedural advisers. In that role, they advise complainants about formulating a complaint, or respondents about responding. They advise about NZAC's process, but do not act in a counselling or advocacy role. After the process has been completed, the procedural advisor is available to act in a debriefing role. Confidentiality is maintained with the person they are advising, within the limitations provided for by the *Code of Ethics*.

STAGES OF THE REP

1. Preparation for a meeting with the complainant and the respondent

When a complaint is assigned to a RET, a case manager is appointed to coordinate the response. A two-member team read the written material provided by both parties and confirm that there is no conflict of interest for them. They formulate initial questions in preparation for separate meetings with the complainant and the respondent. Whenever possible, the supervisor of the respondent is invited to be involved. Only the case manager is in contact with the parties prior to the meeting.

2. Meeting with the complainant

The complainant is invited to meet with the two members of the RET at a mutually acceptable venue, and to bring a support person. The complainant is acknowledged for bringing their concerns to the association's attention and is assured that the matter will be investigated. The complainant's hopes and expectations are discussed, and possible outcomes outlined. Support persons are given an opportunity to speak at the end of the meeting. RET members usually take notes as they hear the complainant's account. Most meetings last about two hours.

3. Meeting with the respondent

This meeting is scheduled on the same day or as soon as possible after the meeting with the complainant. The respondent is encouraged to bring their supervisor to meet with the two members of the RET. Whenever possible, a letter is sent to the supervisor before the interview, outlining how the supervisor can contribute to the process. At least two hours is allowed for the meeting.

The meeting is conducted in three stages, with an opportunity for reflection between each. The RET members:

- hear the respondent's account and responses to questions from the RET;
- identify any concerns the RET members hold about professional behaviour or practice;
- determine any educative and/or remedial action required of the counsellor, and the time frame for that action.

The meeting provides an opportunity for the respondent to describe to the RET their understanding of what happened. The RET members ask about the circumstances that led to the complaint, and, where appropriate, invite the respondent to reflect on and review their practice. The RET then formulates optimal outcomes and discusses them with the respondent and their supervisor. The case manager may set specific tasks with a time frame for completion.

4. Possible outcomes from the RET meetings with the parties

The RET may:

- take no further action;
- facilitate private resolution between the parties;
- identify any restorative or educative steps the RET requires the respondent to take, such as acknowledgment of wrong doing, further professional education or remedial action, specialist consultation to be undertaken, or additional supervision;
- refer the matter back to the IAG, recommending further investigation or a hearing.

5. After the meetings

The case manager writes to the respondent and to the ethics secretary with specific details of the tasks to be undertaken, and the time frame. The complainant is informed, in general terms, of the outcome. They are also later informed when the respondent has satisfied the RET requirements.

RECORDS

The case manager completes an evaluation form to support RET learning and ongoing refinement of the process. Copies of relevant documents are retained by the ethics secretary.

PARTICIPANT FEEDBACK

Feedback from complainants, respondents and supervisors contributes to the ongoing refinement of the REP. My experience has been that these refinements have led to increasing satisfaction with the process and its outcomes. From a complainant's perspective, satisfaction appears to relate to the timeliness of the process, and the opportunity to meet, face to face, with RET members as representatives of NZAC.

RESPONDENTS

Experience indicates that respondents in the REP have offered responses across a continuum, from satisfactory to less satisfactory, to NZAC's requirement that they participate in this process. Most satisfying, from an ethics committee/RET perspective, are those situations where the separate conversations with the parties produce a shared understanding of what has gone wrong; and when, out of this understanding, a respondent and their supervisor then address the ethical practice concerns and provide a written report demonstrating learning. The following excerpt, printed with a respondent's informed consent, is from their written reflections after participating in a REP.[1]

> I can't say enough how valuable this process has been – at the time I wanted the ground to open up and swallow me into a big hole. Having a complaint against me was my worst nightmare coming true. When we had finished the panel interview with you I was pretty gobsmacked as I thought you had been 'tough'. I felt you had been hard on me.
>
> Upon reflection I can see why you were so concerned. I had missed vital, important steps ... The insights gained and lessons learned here, I believe, have stood me in a safer place to practice for myself and my clients. I now have a strong voice in terms of ethical practice in my agency and am willing to stand strong and use the word, "No," to uphold our *Code of Ethics*. In the past I have had a sense of our *Code of Ethics* but had not adhered to them. I now know how important and vital it is that

1 My thanks to the NZAC member who contributed this. Authorship of the contribution is anonymous in order to protect the member's privacy.

I adhere to them and know them and revisit them when I am unsure in my practice.

SUPERVISORS

Anecdotal experience suggests that the degree of involvement of a supervisor is emerging as a critical factor in the REP. When a complaint has been thoroughly explored in supervision prior to the REP meeting, and shortcomings have been identified, it is possible then to have a very rewarding conversation with the respondent about the complainant's experience, and how to improve the respondent's practice. This is when the REP comes into its own, when respondents learn from the experience of a complaint, and, as a result of discussion, reflection and specific tasks, refine their practice to become better counsellors.

CONCLUSION

Given that it often takes courage for a client to formulate a complaint in writing, it has been pleasing to learn that in many instances, clients have experienced some degree of satisfaction after the REP has been completed. Equally, it is encouraging to learn of counsellors who have found the educative tasks set for them to be beneficial to their future practice. Refinement of the REP is ongoing.

PART 6

EXTENDING ETHICS: THE FUTURE IS ALREADY AT HAND

EXTENDING ETHICS: THE FUTURE IS ALREADY AT HAND

Sue Cornforth

Contributions to this book evidence the wide range of interest in ethical praxis amongst NZAC members. The number of contributing authors shows that counsellors are prepared to continue the conversations that have accompanied the development and revisions of NZAC ethical codes, at each successive step. This multi-vocal effort, involving 29 different contributors, further evidences the membership's commitment to the relatively new ethical value of partnership, and can be seen in the amount of co-authoring, the process of review and ongoing commentary, and the various discussions that went into the making of this book. In a sense, this commitment to partnership, to ongoing collegial discussion and working together, is what characterises counselling in New Zealand and makes it unique. This commitment positions local counsellors well in facing the challenges of the future – both those that might be anticipated and those we cannot foresee. This final section aims to extend these ethical conversations by considering how they might proceed in the next few decades, in a globalised and environmentally challenged world – one that increasingly affects what might be thought of as the private space of the counselling room.

The contemporary world is very different from the one in which the talking cures emerged. Three of the main physical markers of the 21st century are the interchange of economies; the movement of peoples; and climate change. Accompanying these material indicators of a rapidly changing world are many other social changes: competition for resources; the development of a knowledge economy in which "people see knowledge in economic terms, as the primary source of all future economic growth" (Gilbert, 2005); new managerialism and tighter structures of accountability, sometimes called neoliberal calculative regimes (see for example, Peters, Marshall & Webster, 1996); more natural disasters as the effects of climate change are increasingly felt (Intergovernmental Panel on Climate Change [IPCC], 2007); fundamentalism of various kinds; older and larger populations; terrorism, and so on. Since the consequences of these changes impact upon every aspect of life, they are counselling concerns and demand ethical attention (American Psychological Association, 2009). However, they make promoting "the safety and well-being of individuals, families, communities, whanau, hapu and iwi" (NZAC, 2002) a daunting task. They raise new questions about the nature of social justice (3.6), and the commitment to do no harm (4.2).

Although the interchange of economies, the movement of peoples, and climate change are interrelated, the two former are commonly referred to as globalisation, while climate change and global warming are often framed as environmental concerns. The link between globalisation and environmental concern often escapes scrutiny. A recent issue of the *International Journal for the Advancement of Counselling* placed the two issues side by side in two different papers that considered the relevance for counselling of globalisation (Paredes et al., 2008) and climate change (Cornforth, 2008). However, many writers who are concerned for social justice call for a more intimate connection, arguing that any ethical consideration must accept the interconnection of both globalisation and climate change: under every question of social justice is the more fundamental question of environmental or ecological justice (Furman & Gruenewald, 2004; Hung, 2007).

The growing gap between rich and poor is founded on a culture of exploitation of natural resources, and disrespect for local communities' relationships with their environments. Globalised economies have not prioritised restitution, and the "developed" countries still leave a legacy of environmental degradation in the "underdeveloped" world. Paredes et al. (2008) concluded their paper by acknowledging that "one of the principal criticisms of globalisation is that its social consequences have been unevenly distributed (Stiglitz 2006; World Commission on the Social Dimensions of Globalisation 2004)", (p. 163). Environmentalists are more explicit in quantifying the disproportionate relationship between affluence, the increasing amount of anthropogenic carbon dioxide emissions that are the main contributors to climate change, and the traumatic effects of these emissions experienced by those in the "underdeveloped" world. The IPCC (2007) reported that poor communities can be especially vulnerable. They tend to have more limited adaptive capacity, and are more dependent on climate-sensitive resources such as local water and food supplies.

When this information is taken into account, the concept of not doing harm becomes so complex that it almost loses the possibility of being meaningful. Harm is inherent in Euro-western consumer-dependent lifestyles and, in particular, in the consumption of oil. Nor can a concern for social justice be limited to local or even national communities, since all peoples of the world are interrelated through both global economies and the use of the global commons: air, water, sunshine and access to outdoor spaces. As noted in Part 1 of this book, the Nuremberg Declaration was intended to produce a version of justice that worked for the good of society as a whole, not just for the politically dominant group. As the media daily confront people with images of the victims of both globalisation and environmental disasters, one cannot claim to be ignorant, notwithstanding the media's frequent failure to make connections between suffering and social obligation. However, the very existence of the caring professions is founded on an ethical commitment to the good of society. As the boundaries of this society are continually extended through both globalisation and the shared use of our global commons, for whom shall counsellors "promote justice" (5.2.h), and what does it now mean to "take account of [our] own cultural biases, and seek to limit any harmful impact of these in [our] work with clients"? (5.2.a)

These new and complex global problems are currently concerning ethicists, many of whom pose important questions about the extent of people's ethical responsibilities and the need to think beyond immediate relationships (for example, Benatar, Daar & Singer, 2005). This relatively new line of ethical thought has received great impetus from environmental ethicists. The field of environmental philosophy has grown over the last 25 years (Jamieson, 2008), presenting, as Sterba (2001) noted, one of the major challenges to traditional ethical approaches. The crucial question of sustainability has been pivotal in allowing the problem to be clearly framed. Bosselmann (2001) wrote:

> Fundamentally, the international sustainability debate has its focus around two ethical questions (Bosselmann, 1999). One is concern to intragenerational justice (between North as South, between rich and poor, etc.) and intergenerational justice (towards future generations). The other question is whether sustainability pursues a technocratic or an ecocentric direction. Any attempt to define and operationalise

> sustainability is a (conscious or unconscious) response to such ethical questions. (p. 178)

Is it possible to escape responsibility for further action by arguing that counsellors' prime responsibility is to a particular client? This has been a time-honoured approach to defining therapeutic responsibility. However, reducing ethical obligations to single parties is no longer tenable. As Fisher (2009) has compellingly argued, without reference to either globalisation or climate change, psychologists have wider "ethical obligations to all parties in every case, regardless of the number or the nature of the relationships" (p. 1). This point has certainly been the message of many of the contributors to this book. However, it has become obvious that all peoples of the world have become "parties in every case," in that they are interrelated by way of their connection either through economies or through shared use of our global commons. Even if counsellors were tempted to restrict their responsibilities to their immediate therapeutic relationships, the delayed effects of climate change in particular threaten all members of the next generation, who stand to inherit a severely, and irrevocably, damaged world. This situation brings the problem closer to home and has led some environmental writers to propose an ethic of self-interest (Pittock, 2005) since counsellors' own interests and safety are also at risk.

Extending counsellors' ethical thinking and sensitivity will involve formulating conscious and explicit responses to the following questions: What does it mean to counsel with unborn generations in mind? What does it mean to accept brotherhood and sisterhood with people we have never met? Can the caring professions stand by and wait for science to find a technological fix to problems of human and ecological distress? These are questions that cannot be avoided. They are questions with which many of the helping professions are currently struggling to engage, and which will, in my opinion, increasingly affect the ethical conversations of counsellors both here and around the world.

The NZAC membership is well-positioned to take part in these debates. Especially relevant is the relatively new commitment to partnership and the membership's experiences of the never-smooth road to reconciliation. Partnership, in the form of solidarity, has been heralded as the hope of a more socially just world. Benetar et al. (2005) foreground the health challenges that affect everyone in the current globalised environment and wrote:

> The underlying basis for new threats to health, life, and security is our failure to adequately pursue the values that play an essential role in improving population health locally and globally ... Foremost amongst these is solidarity – without it, we ignore distant indignities, violations of human rights, inequities, deprivation of freedom, undemocratic regimes, and damage to the environment. (p. 0587)

Here "solidarity" is set against "individual freedom" or autonomy. In terms of the NZAC *Code of Ethics*, solidarity more closely aligns with partnership, and the frequent use of "working with clients" (for example 5.2.e). Solidarity is linked to an ethic of care by Sevenhuijsen (1998): "care without collective solidarity strengthens the privatization and moralization of care" (p. 147).

Larner and Le Heron (2005), too, took partnership beyond the personal to the organisational. Examining the political context of tertiary-sector reform, they identified a current "third period of neo-liberalism [that] is characterised by a 'partnering' ethos [and a] new emphasis on collaboration" (p. 851). They suggested that this partnering phase is set against the previous phase's emphasis on "calculative practices" and accountability (p. 858). Counselling in New Zealand is also affected by these neo-liberal forces, and stands poised at this intersection. Where it goes in the future will depend on what the membership of the profession chooses to prioritise. If a regime of accountability continues to dominate, counsellors' ethical focus is likely to be more restricted to the immediate; if the commitment to partnership continues to grow, there will likely be exciting new developments in the future which will move the profession's focus beyond the local and immediate into the global arena.

Many of the following counselling initiatives are already in place, either in New Zealand or elsewhere in the world, and the possibilities of the future are limited only by our imaginations.

Many counselling organisations and institutions are working to produce a more globalised profession, including possibilities for international accrediting (Paredes et al., 2008). Some have established disaster relief or follow-up response teams ready to respond to international humanitarian and ecological disasters (see, for example, the Dulwich Centre's current projects: http://www.dulwichcentre.com.au/current-projects.html). Some support the development of context-appropriate counselling training/professional education programmes in particular places (Sliep & Kotze, 2007). Some are beginning to write environmental responsibility and a wider version of social justice into their ethical codes: *Counselling, Psychotherapy and Health*, the official research journal of the Australian Counselling Association, includes "respect for ecosystems including planetary, [and] local environments" in its core values. Some are foregrounding globalisation and environmentalism in their training and professional development programmes (for example, British Association for Counselling and Psychotherapy, 2005).

Perhaps the greatest challenge remains in the version of ethics counsellors choose to perpetuate. Many ethicists who centralise globalisation and climate change argue that the main barrier to a more just world is the anthropocentric nature of our ethical awareness (Furman & Gruenewald, 2004; Hung, 2007; Naess, 1984; O'Neill, Holland & Light, 2008). These writers argue that we have gone too far in supporting a view of being human that separates and elevates humankind from the rest of the world, leaving other species and the environment as a resource to be managed, and resulting in an insidious form of "specieism" (Singer, 2002). An alternative perspective foregrounding the human-nature link was first articulated by social psychologists such as Shepard (1982) who coined the term "ecopsychology." This earlier group of psychologists located their concerns within a wider discourse of ecocentric, ontological spirituality, and "deep ecology" (Naess, 1973). Arguing that human well-being is deeply interconnected with the health of the planet, writers such as Fisher (2002), Metzner (1999) and Rozak (1999), each drew on slightly different psychological approaches to explain the difficulty for many people in recognising the importance of this interconnection.

Again the value of partnership may position counsellors in New Zealand well to deal with this challenge. The impetus for the uptake of this value has emerged out of growing Pākehā respect for Māori as Treaty of Waitangi partners, and increasing commitment to the principles of the Treaty, including respect for those tāonga valued by tāngata whenua. In offering themselves for partnership, Pākehā also have knowledge traditions that focus on care for the natural environment. An example is Leopold's (1949) foundational and resilient land ethic, positing that the natural environment has intrinsic value. He left these words, a challenge from the past for the future, which might bring together both tāngata whenua and tauiwi aspirations for care:

> A thing is right when it tends to preserve the integrity, stability, and beauty of the biotic community. It is wrong when it does otherwise. (Leopold, 1949, p. 262)

REFERENCES

PART 1: SITUATING COUNSELLING ETHICS IN AOTEAROA NEW ZEALAND

1.1 ETHICS AS EVERYDAY PRACTICE

Bauman, Z. (1998). What prospects of morality in times of uncertainty? *Theory, Culture & Society, 15*(1), 11–22.

Bauman, Z. (2000). Am I my brother's keeper? *European Journal of Social Work, 3*(1), 5–11.

Beauchamp, T. L. & Childress, J. F. (2009). *Principles of biomedical ethics* (6th ed.). New York: Oxford University Press.

Broverman, I. K., Broverman, D. M., Clarkson, F. E., Rosenkrantz, P. S. & Vogel, S. R. (1970). Sex-role stereotypes and clinical judgments of mental health. *Journal of Consulting and Clinical Psychology, 34*(1), 1–7.

Enns, C. Z. (1993). Twenty years of feminist counseling and therapy: From naming biases to implementing multifaceted practice. *The Counseling Psychologist, 21*(1), 3–87.

Foucault, M. (1988). The ethic of care for the self as a practice of freedom. In J. Bernauer & D. Rasmussen (Eds.), J. D. Gauthier (Tran.), *The final Foucault.* Cambridge, MA: MIT Press.

Gilligan, C. (1982). *In a different voice: Psychological theory and women's development.* Cambridge, MA: Harvard University Press.

Hugman, R. (2005a). *New approaches in ethics for the caring professions.* Basingstoke, United Kingdom: Palgrave Macmillan.

Hugman, R. (2005b). *New approaches in ethics for the caring professions.* Basingstoke, United Kingdom: Palgrave Macmillan.

Levinas, E. (1989). *The Levinas reader.* (S. Hand, Ed.). Malden, MA: Wiley-Blackwell.

Loewenthal, D. & Snell, R. (2001). Psychotherapy as the practice of ethics. In F. P. Barnes & L. Murdin (Eds.), *Values and ethics in the practice of psychotherapy and counselling* (pp. 23–31). Buckingham, United Kingdom: Open University Press.

Ludbrook, R. (2003). *Counselling and the law*. Hamilton, New Zealand: New Zealand Association of Counsellors.

New Zealand Association of Counsellors. (2002). *Code of ethics*. Hamilton, New Zealand: Author.

Nussbaum, M. (2009). Compassion: The basic social emotion. *Social Philosophy and Policy, 13*(01), 27–58.

Sevenhuijsen, S. (2003). The place of care: The relevance of the feminist ethic of care for social policy. *Feminist Theory*, 4(2), 179–197.

Waldegrave, C. (1990). Just therapy. *Dulwich Centre Newsletter, 1*, 5–47.

Welch, S. D. (1990). *A feminist ethic of risk*. Minneapolis, MN: Fortress.

Welfel, E. R. (2006). *Ethics in counseling and psychotherapy: Standards, research, and emerging issues* (3rd ed.). Belmont, CA: Brooks/Cole-Thomson Learning.

Winslade, J. (2002). Presenting the new Code of Ethics. *New Zealand Association of Counsellors' Newsletter*, 23(1), 15–23.

1.2 TE TIRITI AND ETHICS AS DIALOGUE: A UNIQUE CALL TO PARTNERSHIP

Crocket, A. (2009). Interpreting "partnership" as a core value: Some implications of the Treaty of Waitangi for the NZAC Code of Ethics. *New Zealand Journal of Counselling*, 29(2), 61–72.

Royal Commission on Social Policy. (1988). *The April report (Vol. 2)*. Wellington, New Zealand: Author.

Te Wiata, J. (2006). A local Aotearoa New Zealand investigation of the contribution of Maori cultural knowledges to Pakeha identiy and counselling practices. (Master's thesis, University of Waikato, Hamilton, New Zealand). Retrieved from http://hdl.handle.net/10289/2339

Tomm, K. (1993). The ethics of dual relationships. *Dulwich Centre Newsletter*, (2 & 3), 47–54.

1.2b A second reflection on Te Tiriti and ethics as dialogue: A unique call to partnership?

Pere, R. (1982). *Ako: Concepts and learning in the Maori tradition (Working Paper No. 17)*. Hamilton, New Zealand: University of Waikato.

Royal, C. (Ed.). (2003). *The woven universe: Selected writings of Rev. Māori Marsden*. Masterton, New Zealand: The Estate of Rev. Māori Marsden.

Royal, C. (2009). *Mātauranga Māori: An Introduction. (Monograph One)*. Porirua, New Zealand: Mauriora-ki-te-Ao/Living Universe.

1.3 CULTURE IS ALWAYS PRESENT: A CONVERSATION ABOUT ETHICS

Abu-Lughod, L. (2006). Writing against culture. In E. Lewin (Ed.), *Feminist anthropology: A reader* (pp. 153–169). Malden, MA: Blackwell.

Bell, A. (2008). Recognition or ethics? *Cultural Studies*, 22(6), 850–869.

Benhabib, S. (2002). *The claims of culture*. Princeton, NJ: Princeton University Press.

Burman, E. (2004). From difference to intersectionality: Challenges and resources. *European Journal of Psychotherapy, Counselling & Health, 6*(4), 293–308.

Culbertson, P. & Agee, M. (2007). "What's so 'identity' about that word?" *New Zealand Journal of Counselling*, 27(2), 77–95.

Monk, G., Winslade, J. & Sinclair, S. (2008). *New horizons in multicultural counseling: New directions for working with diversity*. Thousand Oaks, CA: Sage.

New Zealand Association of Counsellors. (2002). *Code of ethics*. Hamilton, New Zealand: Author.

Phillips, A. (2007). *Multiculturalism without culture*. Princeton, NJ: Princeton University Press.

1.4 SITUATING ETHICAL PRACTICE IN PHILOSOPHICAL STORYLINES

Axten, D. (2004). The development of supervision ethics. In M. McMahon & W. Patton (Eds.) *Supervision in the helping professions: A practical approach* (pp. 105–116). Frenchs Forest, NSW, Australia: Prentice Hall.

Barnes, F. P. & Murdin, L. (Eds.). (2001). *Values and ethics in the practice of psychotherapy and counselling*. Buckingham, United Kingdom: Open University Press.

Beauchamp, T. & Childress, J. F. (1994). *Principles of biomedical ethics* (4th ed.). New York: Oxford University Press.

Beauchamp, T. L. & Childress, J. F. (2009). *Principles of biomedical ethics* (6th ed.). New York: Oxford University Press.

Belmont Report. (1979).

Bondi, L. (1993). Locating identity politics. In M. Keith & S. Pile (Eds.), *Place and the politics of identity* (pp. 84–101). London, United Kingdom: Routledge.

Chantler, K. (2005). From disconnection to connection: 'Race', gender and the politics of therapy. *British Journal of Guidance & Counselling*, 33(2), 239–256.

Corey, G., Corey, M. S. & Callanan, P. (2007). *Issues and ethics in the helping professions* (7th ed.). Belmont, CA: Thomson Brooks/Cole.

Crocket, A. (2009). Interpreting "partnership" as a core value: Some implications of the Treaty of Waitangi for the NZAC Code of Ethics. *New Zealand Journal of Counselling, 29*(2), 61–72.

D'Cruz, H., Gillingham, P. & Melendez, S. (2007). Reflexivity, its meanings and relevance for social work: A critical review of the literature. *British Journal of Social Work, 37*, 73–90.

Doherty, W. J. (1995). *Soul searching: Why psychotherapy must promote moral responsibility*. New York: Basic Books.

Fairclough, N. (1992). *Discourse and social change*. Cambridge, United Kingdom: Polity.

Fisher, C. & Anushko, A. (2008). Research ethics in social science. In P. Alasuutari, L. Bickman & J. Brannen (Eds.), *The Sage handbook of social research methods* (pp. 95–109). Thousand Oaks, CA: Sage.

Gallagher, M. (2009). Ethics. In E. K. Tisdall, J. Davis, J. M. Davis & M. Gallagher (Eds.), *Researching with children and young people: Research design, methods and analysis* (pp. 11–65). Thousand Oaks, CA: Sage.

Gilligan, C. (1982). *In a different voice: Psychological theory and women's development*. Cambridge, MA: Harvard University Press.

Greig, A. D., Taylor, J. & MacKay, T. (2007). Ethics of doing research with children. In A. D. Greig, J. Taylor & T. MacKay (Eds.), *Doing research with children* (2nd ed., pp. 168–181). London, United Kingdom: Sage.

Hobbes, T. (1651/1994). Leviathan. In P. Singer (Ed.), *Ethics* (pp. 29–35). Oxford, United Kingdom: Oxford University Press.

Hugman, R. (2005). *New approaches in ethics for the caring professions*. Basingstoke: Palgrave Macmillan.

Hume, D. (1739). Reason and passion. In *Ethics* (pp. 118–123). Oxford, United Kingdom: Oxford University Press.

Kitchener, K. S. (1984). Intuition, critical evaluation and ethical principles: The foundation for ethical decisions in counseling psychology. *The Counseling Psychologist, 12*(3), 43–55.

Levinas, E. (1989). *The Levinas reader*. (S. Hand, Ed.). Malden, MA: Wiley-Blackwell.

Locke, J. (1690). *Two treatises of government: A critical edition with an introduction and apparatus criticus by Peter Laslett*. Cambridge, United Kingdom: Cambridge University Press.

Neiman, S. (2002). *Evil in modern thought*. Princeton, NJ: Princeton University Press.

New Zealand Association of Counsellors. (1991). *Code of ethics*. Author, Hamilton, New Zealand: Author.

New Zealand Association of Counsellors. (2002). *Code of ethics*. Author, Hamilton, New Zealand: Author.

Nussbaum, M. C. (1992). Human functioning and social justice: In defense of Aristotelian essentialism. *Theory, 20*(2), 202–246.

Paredes, D. M., Choi, K. M., Dipal, M., Edwards-Joseph, A. R., Ermakov, N., Gouveia, A. T., Jain, S., et al. (2008). Globalization: A brief primer for counsellors. *International Journal for the Advancement of Counselling, 30*(3), 155–166.

Rhodes, R. (2005). Rethinking research ethics. *The American Journal of Bioethics, 5*(1), 7–28.

Rogers, C. R. (1962). The interpersonal relationship: The core of guidance. *Harvard Educational Review, 32*(4), 416–429.

Rossiter, A., Prilleltensky, I. & Walsh-Bowers, R. (2000). A postmodern perspective on professional ethics. In B. Fawcett, B. Featherstone, J. Fook & A. Rossiter (Eds.), *Practice and research in social work: Postmodern feminist perspectives* (pp. 83–103). London: Routledge.

Rousseau, J. J. (1762). The social contract. In R. Solomon (Ed.), *Introducing philosophy: A text with integrated readings* (6th ed., pp. 635–639). London, United Kingdom: Routledge.

Small, R. (2008). Teaching, professionalism and ethics. In V. M. Carpenter, J. Jesson, P. Roberts & M. Stephenson (Eds.), *Nga kaupapa here: Connections and contradictions in eduation* (pp. 57–65). Melbourne, Australia: Cengage Learning.

The Declaration of Helsinki. (1964).

The Geneva Convention. (1949).

Waldegrave, C. (1990). Just therapy. *Dulwich Centre Newsletter, 1*, 5–47.

Webb, S. (1998). New Zealand Association of Counsellors: Helping to make a difference. *New Zealand Journal of Counselling, 19*(1 & 2), 67–78.

Winslade, J. (2002). Presenting the new Code of Ethics. *New Zealand Association of Counsellors' Newsletter, 23*(1), 15–23.

Further reading

Hugman, R. (2003). Professional values and ethics in social work: Reconsidering postmodernism? *British Journal of Social Work, 33*(8), 1025–1041.

1.5 MAKING DECISIONS FOR ETHICAL ACTION

Bond, T. (2010). *Standards and ethics for counselling in action* (3rd ed.). London, United Kingdom: Sage.

Cottone, R. R. (2001). A social constructivism model of ethical decision making in counseling. *Journal of Counseling & Development, 79*(1), 39–45.

Cottone, R. R. (2004). Displacing the psychology of the individual in ethical decision-making: The social constructivism model. *Canadian Journal of Counselling/Revue Canadienne de Counseling, 38*(1), 5–13.

Cottone, R. R. & Claus, R. E. (2000). Ethical decision-making models: A review of the literature. *Journal of Counseling & Development, 78*(3), 275–283.

Hawkins, A. H. (1997). Medical ethics and the epiphanic dimension of narrative. In H. L. Nelson (Ed.), *Stories and their limits: Narrative approaches to bioethics* (pp. 153–170). New York: Routledge.
Hill, M., Glaser, K. & Harden, J. (1998). A feminist model for ethical decision making. *Women & Therapy, 21*(3), 101–121.
Ludbrook, R. (2003). *Counselling and the law*. Hamilton, New Zealand: New Zealand Association of Counsellors.
New Zealand Association of Counsellors. (2002). *Code of ethics*. Hamilton, New Zealand: Author.
Rossiter, A., Prilleltensky, I. & Walsh-Bowers, R. (2000). A postmodern perspective on professional ethics. In B. Fawcett, B. Featherstone, J. Fook & A. Rossiter (Eds.), *Practice and research in social work: Postmodern feminist perspectives* (pp. 83–103). London, United Kingdom: Routledge.
The Privacy Act. (1993).
Walden, S. L. (2006). Inclusion of the client perspective in ethical practice. In B. Herlihy & G. Corey (Eds.), *Boundary issues in counseling: Multiple roles and responsibilities* (2nd ed., pp. 40–47). Alexandria, VA: American Counseling Association.

1.6 USING A CODE OF ETHICS AS A WORKING DOCUMENT

Hugman, R. (2005). *New approaches in ethics for the caring professions*. Basingstoke, United Kingdom: Palgrave Macmillan.
New Zealand Association of Counsellors. (2002). *Code of ethics*. Hamilton, New Zealand: Author.
Winslade, J. (2002). Presenting the new Code of Ethics. *New Zealand Association of Counsellors' Newsletter, 23*(1), 15–23.

PART 2: PRESENTING OURSELVES AS PROFESSIONALS

2.1 MARKETING, ADVERTISING AND ETHICS: COMMUNICATING WITH THE PUBLIC

American Counseling Association. (2005). Code of Ethics. Retrieved from www.counseling.org
Davis, J. & Freeman, M. (1996). *Marketing for therapists: A handbook for success in managed care*. San Francisco, CA: Jossey-Bass.
Kotler, P. & Bloom, P. N. (1984). *Marketing professional services*. Englewood Cliffs, NJ: Prentice-Hall.
Leicht, K. T. & Fennell, M. L. (2001). *Professional work: A sociological approach*. Malden, MA: Wiley-Blackwell.

Lovelock, C. H., Patterson, P. G. & Walker, R. H. (1998). *Services marketing: Australia and New Zealand*. Sydney, Australia: Prentice Hall.
Manthei, R. & Miller, J. (2000). *Good counselling: A guide for clients*. Auckland, New Zealand: Pearson.
Miller, J. H. (2003). Marketing counselling in New Zealand: The images of practice. *New Zealand Journal of Counselling, 24*(1), 66–82.
New Zealand Association of Counsellors. (2002). *Code of ethics*. Hamilton, New Zealand: Author.
New Zealand Association of Psychotherapists. (2008). Code of ethics. Retrieved from http://nzap.org.nz/about/code-of-ethics
New Zealand Psychological Society. (2002). The code of ethics for psychologists working in Aotearoa/New Zealand. Retrieved from http://www.psychology.org.nz/Code_of_Ethics

2.2 PROFESSIONAL DISCLOSURE STATEMENTS

Coles, D. (1995). A pilot use of letters to clients before the initial session. *Australian and New Zealand Journal of Family Therapy, 16*(4), 209–213.
Gill, S. J. (1982). Professional disclosure and consumer protection in counseling. *Personnel and Guidance Journal, 60*(7), 443–446.
Miller, J. H. (2003). Marketing counselling in New Zealand: The images of practice. *New Zealand Journal of Counselling, 24*(1), 66–82.

2.3 THE SETTING FOR COUNSELLING: PRIVATE PRACTICE

Cornforth, S. & Sewell, S. (2004). Where have they gone? What are they doing? The profiles and destinations of counselling graduates, 1997–2002. *New Zealand Journal of Counselling, 25*(1), 31–47.
Manthei, R. J., Rich, P., Agee, M., Monk, G., Miller, J., Bunce, J., Webb, S., et al. (1994). Being in control: A survey of counsellors who have moved into private practice. *New Zealand Journal of Counselling, 16*(2), 14–31.
New Zealand Association of Counsellors. (2002). *Code of ethics*. Hamilton, New Zealand: Author.
New Zealand Association of Counsellors. (2010). Registration survey of members. Hamilton, New Zealand: Author.
Paton, I. (1995). Perils and pleasures of private practice: An update. *New Zealand Journal of Counselling, 17*(2), 45–1.
Paton, I. (1999). The nature and experience of private practice in New Zealand. *New Zealand Journal of Counselling, 20*(1), 1–3.
Paton, I. (2005). How to have your cake and eat it too: Counselling in private practice from home. *New Zealand Journal of Counselling, 26*(2), 55–9.
Syme, G. (1994). *Counselling in independent practice*. Buckingham, United Kingdom: Open University Press.

2.4 WORKING BEYOND THE AGENCY WALLS

Crocket, K. (2008). Narrative therapy. In J. Frew & M. Spiegler (Eds.), *Contemporary psychotherapies for a diverse world* (pp. 489-531). Boston, MA: Houghton Mifflin.

Epston, D., White, M. & "Ben." (1995). Consulting your consultants: A means to the co-construction of alternative knowledges. In S. Friedman (Ed.), *The reflecting team in action: Collaborative practice in family therapy* (pp. 277–313). New York: Guilford Press.

Hare-Mustin, R. (1994). Discourses in the mirrored room: A postmodern analysis of therapy. *Family Process, 33*(3), 19–35.

New Zealand Association of Counsellors. (2002). *Code of ethics*. Hamilton, New Zealand: Author.

Waldegrave, C. (1990). Just therapy. *Dulwich Centre Newsletter, 1*, 5–47.

White, M. & Epston, D. (1990). *Narrative means to therapeutic ends*. New York: Norton.

Further reading

Madsen, W. C. (2007). *Collaborative therapy with multi-stressed families* (2nd ed.). New York: Guilford Press.

2.5 SOLICITING CLIENTS

New Zealand Association of Counsellors. (2002). *Code of ethics*. Hamilton, New Zealand: Author.

2.6 TESTIMONIALS FROM CLIENTS

Health Information Privacy Code. (1994).

New Zealand Association of Counsellors. (2002). *Code of ethics*. Hamilton, New Zealand: Author.

Winslade, J. (1998). Soliciting references from clients. *New Zealand Association of Counsellors' Newsletter, 19*(1), 21–23.

2.7 ETHICS FOR RESEARCH AND PUBLICATION

Bond, T. (2004). Ethical guidelines for researching counselling and psychotherapy. *Counselling and Psychotherapy Research, 4*(2), 10–19.

Chantler, K. & Smailes, S. (2004). Working with differences: Issues for research and counselling practice. *Counselling and Psychotherapy Research, 4*(2), 34–39.

Cornforth, S. (2006). *Controversies in counselling: Rethinking therapy's ethical base*. Unpublished doctoral dissertation, Victoria University of Wellington, New Zealand.

Crocket, K. (2004). From narrative practice in counselling to narrative practice in research: A professional identity story. *International Journal of Narrative Therapy and Community Work, 2*, 64–67.

Crocket, K., Pentecost, M., Cresswell, R., Paice, C., Tollestrup, D., de Vries, M. & Wolfe, R. (2009). Informing supervision practice through research: A narrative inquiry. *Counselling and Psychotherapy Research, 9*(2), 101–107.

Denzin, N. K. & Lincoln, Y. S. (2005). *The Sage handbook of qualitative research* (3rd ed.). Thousand Oaks, CA: Sage.

Etherington, K. (1996). The counsellor as researcher: Boundary issues and critical dilemmas. *British Journal of Guidance & Counselling, 24*(3), 339–346.

Feltham, C. (2002). *What's the good of counselling and psychotherapy? The benefits explained.* London, United Kingdom: Sage.

Haraway, D. (1988). Situated knowledges: The science question in feminism as a site of discourse on the privilege of partial perspective. *Feminist Studies, 14*, 575–599.

Kendall, M. G. & Buckland, W. R. (1975). *A dictionary of statistical terms.* Essex, United Kingdom: Longman.

Lincoln, Y. S. & Denzin, N. K. (2005). Epilogue: The eighth and ninth moments: Qualitative research in/and the fractured future. In N. K. Denzin & Y. S. Lincoln (Eds.). *The Sage handbook of qualitative research* (3rd ed.) (pp. 1115–1126). Thousand Oaks, CA: Sage.

Manthei, R. (2006). Clients talk about their experience of seeking counselling. *British Journal of Guidance & Counselling, 34*(4), 519–538.

McLeod, J. (2003). *Doing counselling research* (2nd ed.). London, United Kingdom: Sage.

McLeod, J. (2004). Changing the landscape through research: What you can do to make a difference. *Healthcare Counselling and Psychotherapy Journal, 4*(4), 3–6.

New Zealand Association of Counsellors. (2002). *Code of ethics.* Hamilton, New Zealand: Author.

Pettifer, M. (2003). Generating a research prioroty consensus: A Delphi exercise. *Healthcare Counselling and Psychotherapy Journal, 3*(1), 5–7.

Scheurich, J. J. (1997). *Research method in the postmodern.* London, United Kingdom: The Falmer Press.

Smith, L. T. (1999). *Decolonising methodologies: Research and indigenous peoples.* Dunedin, New Zealand: University of Otago Press.

Speedy, J. (2004). Living a more peopled life: Definitional ceremony as inquiry into psychotherapy 'outcomes'. *International Journal of Narrative Therapy & Community Work, 3*, 43–53.

Sterba, J. P. (2001). *Three challenges to ethics.* New York: Oxford University Press.

Vallance, K. (2004). Exploring counsellor perceptions of the impact of counselling supervision on clients. *British Journal of Guidance & Counselling, 32*(4), 559–574.
Weedon, C. (1987). *Feminist practice and poststructuralist theory*. Oxford, United Kingdom: Blackwell.
Wild, C. J. & Seber, G. A. (2000). *Chance encounters: A first course in data analysis and inference.* New York: John Wiley & Sons.
Willig, C. (2001). *Introducing qualitative research in psychology: Adventures in theory and method.* Buckingham, United Kingdom: Open University Press.

Further reading

Agee, M., Culbertson, P. & Mariu, L. (2005). A bibliography of literature related to Maori mental health. *New Zealand Journal of Counselling, 26*(2), 1–37.
American Psychological Association (2001). *Publication Manual of the American Psychological Association* (5th ed.). Washington, D.C: Author.
Crocket, K. (2004). From narrative practice in counselling to narrative practice in research: A professional identity story. *The International Journal of Narrative Therapy and Community Work,* (2), 63–67.
Manthei, R. (2001). Content analysis of the *New Zealand Journal of Counselling*: Volumes 13–21, 1991–2000. *New Zealand Journal of Counselling, 22*(1), 1-12.
Manthei, R. & Miller, J. (2001). New Zealand counselling, therapy and guidance-related literature published between 1990 and 1999: A bibliography. *New Zealand Journal of Counselling, 22*(1), 13–110.

PART 3: SOME PRAGMATICS FOR PRACTICE

3.1 A FEW NOTES ABOUT NOTES

Cornforth, S. (2006). A discursive approach to the registration debate. *New Zealand Journal of Counselling, 26*(3), 1–15.
Ludbrook, R. (2003). *Counselling and the law.* Hamilton, New Zealand: New Zealand Association of Counsellors.
Manthei, R. (2008). Response to the special registration newsletter April 2008. *Newsletter of the New Zealand Association of Counsellors, 29*(1), 21–23.
New Zealand Association of Counsellors. (2008). *Special registration newsletter.* Hamilton, New Zealand: Author.
NZ Mental Health Commission. (2006). Retrieved from http://www.mhc.govt.nz/Content/FAQ/Privacy-Issues.htm
New Zealand Association of Counsellors. (2002). *Code of ethics.* Hamilton, New Zealand: Author.

Relevant Law

Accident Compensation Corporation Act 2001
Health Information Privacy Code 1994
Health Practitioners Competence Assurance Act 2006
Health (Retention of Health Information) Regulations 1996
Guidance Material for Health Practitioners on Mental Health Information – Privacy Commissioner
Official Information Act 1982
Privacy Act 1993

3.2 MORE NOTES ABOUT NOTES

Health Information Privacy Code 1994
Ludbrook, R. (2003). *Counselling and the law*. Hamilton, New Zealand: New Zealand Association of Counsellors.
New Zealand Association of Counsellors. (2002). *Code of ethics*. Hamilton, New Zealand: Author.

Relevant Law

Children, Young Persons and their Families Act 1989
Children and Young Persons Act 2008
Contraception, Sterilisation and Abortion Act 1977
Mental Health Act 1992
New Zealand Public Health and Disability Act 2000

3.3 SCHOOL COUNSELLORS: CLIENTS, COLLEAGUES AND CONFIDENTIALITY

Agee, M. N. (1997). Privacy and the school counsellor. *Access: Critical Perspectives on Cultural* and *Policy Studies in Education, 16*(1), 20–36.
Daly, M. & Holden, L. (1986). *Youth and the law*. Wellington, New Zealand: Research Unit, Dept. of Internal Affairs.
Hawkins, H. & Monk, G. (1995). School counselling: An ethical minefield? *NZ Journal of Counselling, 17*(1), 1–7.
Ludbrook, R. (2003). *Counselling* and *the law*. Hamilton, New Zealand: New Zealand Association of Counsellors.
New Zealand Association of Counsellors. (2002). *Code of ethics*. Hamilton, New Zealand: Author.
Post Primary Teachers' Association & New Zealand Association of Counsellors. (2010). The school guidance counsellor: Guidelines for principals, boards of trustees, teachers and guidance counsellors, retrieved 9 July 2010 from http://www.nzac.org.nz/schoolguidancecounsellorappointmentkit.html

Winslade, J. (2002). Presenting the new Code of Ethics. *New Zealand Association of Counsellors' Newsletter*, 23(1), 15–23.

3.4 EVEN-HANDEDNESS IN RELATIONSHIP COUNSELLING

Hendrick, S. (1995). *Close relationships: What couple therapists can learn*. Pacific Grove, CA: Brooks/Cole Publishing.

3.5 EVEN-HANDEDNESS IN RELATIONSHIP COUNSELLING: A COMPANION PIECE

Bird, J. (2004). *Talk that sings: Therapy in a new linguistic key*. Auckland, New Zealand: Edge Press.
Bond, T. (2000). *Standards and ethics for counselling in action*. London, United Kingdom: Sage.
Claiborne, L. & Drewery, W. (2010). *Human development: Family, place, culture*. Sydney, Australia: McGraw-Hill.
Fanslow, J. L. & Robinson, E. M. (2004). Violence against women in New Zealand: Prevalence and health consequences. *The New Zealand Medical Journal*. Retrieved from http://www.nzma.org.nz/journal/117-1206/1173/
Fisher, M. A. (2009). Replacing "who is the client?" with a different ethical question. *Professional Psychology: Research and Practice*, 40(1), 1–7.
New Zealand Association of Counsellors. (2002). *Code of ethics*. Hamilton, New Zealand: Author.
White, M. (1986). Couple therapy: Urgency for sameness or appreciation of difference. *Dulwich Centre Review/Summer*, 11–13.

3.6 MULTIPLE RELATIONSHIPS

Campbell, C. D. & Gordon, M. C. (2003). Acknowledging the inevitable: Understanding multiple relationships in rural practice. *Professional Psychology: Research and Practice*, 34(4), 430–434.
Cottone, R. (2005). Detrimental therapist–client relationships: Beyond thinking of "dual" or "multiple" roles: Reflections on the 2001 AAMFT Code of Ethics. *The American Journal of Family Therapy*, 33(1), 1–17.
Durie, M. (1999). Paiheretia: An integrated approach to counselling. *The New Zealand Association of Counsellors Newsletter*, 20(1), 15–22.
Durie, M. (2001). *Mauri ora: The dynamics of Maori health*. Melbourne, Australia: Oxford University Press.
Hill, M. R. & Mamalakis, P. M. (2001). Family therapists and religious communities: Negotiating dual relationships. *Family Relations*, 50(3), 199–208.

Kessler, L. E. & Waehler, C. A. (2005). Addressing multiple relationships between clients and therapists in lesbian, gay, bisexual, and transgender communities. *Professional Psychology: Research and Practice, 36*(1), 66–72.

Lazarus, A. A. & Zur, O. (2002). Introduction. In A. A. Lazarus & O. Zur (Eds.), *Dual relationships and psychotherapy* (pp. xxvii–xxxiii). New York: Springer.

Mattison, D., Jayaratne, S. & Croxton, T. (2002). Client or former client? Implications of ex-client definition on social work practice. *Social work, 47*(1), 55–64.

Mellow, M. (2005). The work of rural professionals: Doing the gemeinschaft-gesellschaft gavotte. *Rural Sociology, 70*, 50–69.

Moleski, S. M. & Kiselica, M. S. (2005). Dual relationships: A continuum ranging from the destructive to the therapeutic. *Journal of Counseling and Development, 83*(1), 3–11.

New Zealand Association of Counsellors. (2002). *Code of ethics*. Hamilton, New Zealand: Author.

Pope, K. S. (1991). Dual relationships in psychotherapy. *Ethics & Behavior, 1*(1), 21–34.

Welfel, E. R. (2010). *Ethics in counselling and psychotherapy: Standards, research, and emerging issues* (4th ed.). Belmont, CA: Brooks/Cole Cengage Learning.

Younggren, J. N. & Gottlieb, M. C. (2004). Managing risk when contemplating multiple relationships. *Professional Psychology: Research and Practice, 35*(3), 255–260.

Zur, O. (2005a). In celebration of dual relationships: How prohibition increases the chance of exploitation or harm. *Psychotherapy in Australia, 12*(1), 36–39.

Zur, O. (2005b). The dumbing down of psychology: Faulty beliefs about boundary crossings and dual relationships. In R. Wright & N. Cummings (Eds.), *Destructive trends in mental health: The well-intentioned path to harm* (pp. 253–282). New York: Brunner-Routledge.

3.7 MANAGING COMPLEX RELATIONSHIPS IN PASTORAL AND CHURCH-BASED COUNSELLING

Claret, M. (2005). 'But it's different in this case': Is there a case for multi-role relationships? *Psychotherapy in Australia, 12*(1), 48–55.

Culbertson, P. L. (2000). *Caring for God's people: Counseling and Christian wholeness*. Minneapolis, MN: Fortress Press.

Culbertson, P. L. & Shippee, A. B. (1990). *The pastor: Readings from the Patristic period*. Minneapolis, MN: Fortress Press.

Doehring, C. (1995). *Taking care. Monitoring power dynamics and relational boundaries in pastoral care and counseling*. Nashville, TN: Abingdon Press.

Haug, I. E. (1999). Boundaries and the use and misuse of power and authority: Ethical complexities for clergy psychotherapists. *Journal of Counseling & Development, 77*(4), 411–17.
Miller, H. M. & Atkinson, D. R. (1988). The clergyperson as counselor: An inherent conflict of interest. *Counseling and Values, 32*(2), 116–123.
New Zealand Association of Counsellors. (2002). *Code of ethics.* Hamilton, New Zealand: Author.
Parent, M. S. (2006). Boundaries and roles in ministry counseling. *American Journal of Pastoral Counseling, 8*(2), 1–25.
Syme, G. (2003). *Dual relationships in counselling and psychotherapy.* London, United Kingdom: Sage.

Further reading

American Association of Pastoral Counselors. (1994). *Code of ethics.* Fairfax, VA: Author. Retrieved October 3, 2007, from http://www.aapc.org/ethics.cfm.
New Zealand Christian Counselling Association. (2001). *Code of Ethics.* Retrieved November 19, 2007, from http://www.nzcca.org.nz.

3.8 MANAGING COMPLEX RELATIONSHIPS RELATIONSHIPS IN LESBIAN, GAY, BISEXUAL, TRANSGENDER AND INTERSEX COMMUNITIES

Gabriel, L. (2005). *Speaking the unspeakable: The ethics of dual relationships in counselling and psychotherapy.* London, United Kingdom: Psychology Press.
Gabriel, L. & Davies, D. (2000). The management of ethical dilemmas associated with dual relationships. In C. Neal & D. Davies (Eds.), *Issues in therapy with lesbian, gay, bisexual, and transgender clients* (pp. 35–54). Buckingham, United Kingdom: Open University Press.
Kessler, L. E. & Waehler, C. A. (2005). Addressing multiple relationships between clients and therapists in lesbian, gay, bisexual, and transgender communities. *Professional Psychology: Research and Practice, 36*(1), 66–72.
New Zealand Association of Counsellors. (2002). *Code of ethics.* Hamilton, New Zealand: Author.
Syme, G. (2003). *Dual relationships in counselling and psychotherapy.* London, United Kingdom: Sage.

3.9 WORKING WITHIN THE SCOPE OF OUR COMPETENCE

Everall, R. D. & Paulson, B. L. (2004). Burnout and secondary traumatic stress: Impact on ethical behaviour. *Canadian Journal of Counselling, 38*(1), 25–35.
Kolb, D. A. (1984). *Experiential learning: Experience as the source of learning and development.* Englewood-Cliffs, NJ: Prentice-Hall.

New Zealand Association of Counsellors. (2002). *Code of ethics*. Hamilton, New Zealand: Author.

Pearlman, L. A. & Saakvitne, K. W. (1995). *Trauma and the therapist*. New York: Norton.

Weingarten, K. (2003). *Common shock: Witnessing violence every day: How we are harmed, how we can heal*. New York: Dutton.

Welfel, E. R. (2010). *Ethics in counselling and psychotherapy: Standards, research, and emerging issues* (4th ed.). Belmont, CA: Brooks/Cole Cengage Learning.

3.10 UNBEARABLE AFFECT IN ETHICAL PROBLEMS

Ferenczi, S. (1955). *Final contributions to the problems and methods of psycho-analysis*. (M. Balint, Ed., E. Mosbacher, Tran.). London, United Kingdom: Hogarth Press.

O'Connor, M. & Macfarlane, A. (2002). New Zealand Maori stories and symbols: Family value lessons for Western counsellors. *International Journal for the Advancement of Counselling, 24*(4), 223–237.

Reed, A. W. (2004). *Reed book of Māori mythology*. (R. Calman, Ed.). Auckland, New Zealand: Reed Publishing.

3.11 PHYSICAL TOUCH IN COUNSELLING RELATIONSHIPS

Hetherington, A. (1998). The use and abuse of touch in therapy and counselling. *Counselling Psychology Quarterly, 11*(4), 361–364.

Hunter, M. & Struve, J. (1998). *The ethical use of touch in psychotherapy*. London, United Kingdom: Sage.

Kitzinger, C. (2000). Doing feminist conversation analysis. *Feminism Psychology, 10*(2), 163–193.

McNeil-Haber, F. M. (2004). Ethical considerations in the use of nonerotic touch in psychotherapy with children. *Ethics & Behavior, 14*(2), 123–140.

New Zealand Association of Counsellors. (2002). *Code of ethics*. Hamilton, New Zealand: Author.

Strozier, A. L., Krizek, C. & Sale, K. (2003). Touch: Its use in psychotherapy. *Journal of Social Work Practice, 17*(1), 49–62.

Tune, D. (2001). Is touch a valid therapeutic intervention? Early returns from a qualitative study of therapists' views. *Counselling and Psychotherapy Research, 1*(3), 167–171.

Tune, D. (2008). How close do I get to my clients? In W. Dryden & A. Reeves (Eds.), *Key issues for counselling in action* (pp. 257–269). London, United Kingdom: Sage.

Welfel, E. R. (2006). *Ethics in counseling and psychotherapy: Standards, research, and emerging issues* (3rd ed.). Belmont, CA: Brooks/Cole-Thomson Learning.

Willison, B. & Masson, R. (1986). The role of touch in therapy: An adjunct to communication. *Journal of Counseling & Development, 64*(8), 497–500.

Winslade, J. & White, C. (2002). An analysis of ethics complaints to NZAC: 1991–2000. *New Zealand Journal of Counselling,* 23(2), 1–13.

Zur, O. & Nordmarken, N. (2006). To touch or not to touch: Rethinking the prohibition on touch in psychotherapy and counseling. ADPTC Newsletter. Retrieved from http://www.aptc.org/news/112006/article_one.html

Further reading

Syme, G. (2003). Touch: Finding the limits (Chapter 5, pp. 55–68). *Dual relationships in counselling and psychotherapy.* London, United Kingdom: Sage.

3.12 WHEN A CLIENT DIES

Agee, M. N. (2001). *Surviving loss by suicide: Counsellors' experience of client suicide.* Unpublished doctoral dissertation, University of Auckland, New Zealand.

Bond, T. (2000). *Standards and ethics for counselling in action.* London, United Kingdom: Sage.

New Zealand Association of Counsellors. (2002). *Code of ethics.* Hamilton, New Zealand: Author.

Rando, T. A. (1993). *Treatment of complicated mourning.* Champaign, IL: Research Press.

3.13 COMMUNICATING WITH OTHER PROFESSIONALS: REFERRAL AND OTHER PRACTICES

Manthei, R. J. (1997). *Counselling: The skills of finding solutions to problems.* Auckland, New Zealand: Longman.

New Zealand Association of Counsellors. (2002). *Code of ethics.* Hamilton, New Zealand: Author.

Simblett, G. J. (1997). Leila and the tiger: Narrative approaches to psychiatry. In G. Monk, J. Winslade, K. Crocket & D. Epston (Eds.), *Narrative therapy in practice: The archaeology of hope* (pp. 121–157). San Francisco: Jossey-Bass.

Further reading

Bentley, K. J., Walsh, J. & Farmer, R. (2005). Referring clients for psychiatric medication: Best practices for social workers. *Best Practices in Mental Health, 1*, 59–71.

Brearley, J. (1995). *Counselling and social work.* Buckingham, United Kingdom: Open University Press.

Rice, N. M. & Follette, V. M. (2003). The termination and referral of clients. In W. O'Donohue & K. Ferguson (Eds.) *Handbook of professional ethics for psychologists: Issues, questions, and controversies* (pp. 147–166). London, United Kingdom: Sage.

Williams, S. (1993). *An incomplete guide to referral issues for counselors.* Manchester, United Kingdom: PCCS Books.

3.14 ONLINE PRACTICES

Evans, J. (2009). *Online counselling and guidance skills: A practical resource for trainees and practitioners.* London, United Kingdom: Sage.

Gackenbach, J. (Ed.). (2007). *Psychology and the internet: Intrapersonal, interpersonal and transpersonal implications.* Burlington, MA: Elsevier/Academic Press.

Jones, G. & Stokes, A. (2008). *Online counselling: A handbook for practitioners.* Basingstoke, United Kingdom: Palgrave Macmillan.

New Zealand Association of Counsellors. (2002). *Code of ethics.* Hamilton, New Zealand: Author.

Wright, J. K. (2007). Online text-based counselling: Reflections of a technophobe. *New Zealand Journal of Counselling, 27*(1), 43–54.

3.15 ELECTRONIC RECORDING OF COUNSELLING CONVERSATIONS

Aveline, M. (1997). The use of audiotapes in supervision of psychotherapy. In G. Shipton (Ed.), *Supervision of psychotherapy and counselling: Making a place to think* (pp. 80–92). Buckingham, United Kingdom: Open University Press.

Crocket, K. (2004). Storying counselors: Producing professional selves in supervision. In D. Pare & G. Larner (Eds.), *Collaborative practice in psychology and therapy* (pp. 171-181). New York: Haworth Press.

Crocket, K., Pentecost, M., Cresswell, R., Paice, C., Tollestrup, D., de Vries, M. & Wolfe, R. (2009). Informing supervision practice through research: A narrative inquiry. *Counselling and Psychotherapy Research, 9*(2), 101–107.

Depree, J. (2009). *Couple counselling.* Paper presented at the New Zealand Association of Counsellors' National Conference, 17–20 September 2009, Hamilton.

Speer, S. & Hutchby, I. (2003). From ethics to analytics: Aspects of participants' orientations to the presence and relevance of recording devices. *Sociology, 37*(2), 315-337.
Sweet, G. (1998). Welcome to the tea party. *New Zealand Association of Counsellors' Newsletter, 18*(4), 27-28.
White, M. (1997). *Narratives of therapists' lives.* Adelaide, Australia: Dulwich.
White, M. (2007). *Maps of narrative practice.* New York: Norton.

3.16 RESPONSIBILITIES TO OTHERS IN A CLIENT'S LIFE

Crocket, K. (2005). Working on fault lines: A perspective on counselling supervision in New Zealand. In L. Beddoe, J. Worral & F. Howard (Eds.). *Weaving together the strands of supervision* (pp. 7–13). Auckland, New Zealand: University of Auckland.
Doherty, W. J. (1995). *Soul searching: Why psychotherapy must promote moral responsibility.* New York: Basic Books.
Fisher, M. A. (2009). Replacing "Who is the client?" with a different ethical question. *Professional Psychology: Research and Practice, 40*(1), 1–7.
Holloway, E. (1995). *Clinical supervision: A systems approach.* Thousand Oaks, CA: Sage.
New Zealand Association of Counsellors. (2002). *Code of ethics.* Hamilton, New Zealand: Author.
Sevenhuijsen, S. (1998). *Citizenship and the ethics of care: Feminist considerations on justice, morality, and politics.* New York: Routledge.

3.17 IMMINENT THREAT OF SERIOUS HARM

Agee, M. N. (2001). *Surviving loss by suicide: Counsellors' experiences of client suicide.* Unpublished doctoral dissertation, University of Auckland, New Zealand.
Bond, T. (2010). *Standards and ethics for counselling in action* (3rd ed.). London, United Kingdom: Sage.
Corey, G., Corey, M. S. & Callanan, P. (2007). *Issues and ethics in the helping professions* (7th ed.). Belmont, CA: Thomson Brooks/Cole.
Granello, D. H. (2010). The process of suicide risk assessment: Twelve core principles. *Journal of Counseling & Development, 88*(3), 363–370.
Ministry of Health. (2008a). *The evidence for action: New Zealand suicide prevention action plan 2008–2012.* Wellington, New Zealand: Author. Retrieved from http://www.moh.govt.nz/moh.nsf/indexmh/nz-suicide-prevention-action-plan-2008–2012
Ministry of Health. (2008b). *The summary for action: New Zealand suicide prevention action plan 2008-2012.* Wellington, New Zealand: Author. Retrieved from http://www.moh.govt.nz/moh.nsf/indexmh/suicideprevention-strategyandplan#plan

New Zealand Association of Counsellors. (2002). *Code of ethics*. Hamilton, New Zealand: Author.

Shallcross, L. (2010). Confronting the threat of suicide. *Counseling Today Online*. Retrieved from http://www.counseling.org/Publications/CounselingTodayArticles.aspx?AGuid=033c7c06-f120-4f44-aa79-b181777d00e7

Further reading

Aveline, M. (2003). Complexities of practice: Psychotherapy in the real world. In F. P. Barnes & L. Murdin (Eds.), *Values and ethics in the practice of psychotherapy and counselling* (pp. 128–143). Buckingham, United Kingdom: Open University Press.

Shillito-Clarke, C. (2000). Question 4: What are my responsibilities when a client's actions or behaviour puts others at risk or when a client is at risk from the behaviour of others? In C. Jones, C. Shillito-Clarke, G. Syme, D. Hill, R. Casemore & L. Murdin, *Questions of ethics in counselling and psychotherapy* (pp. 29–32). Buckingham: Open University Press.

Shillito-Clarke, C. (2000). Question 9: How should I proceed when working with someone who expresses serious suicidal thoughts and feelings? What issues need considering? In C. Jones, C. Shillito-Clarke, G. Syme, D. Hill, R. Casemore & L. Murdin, *Questions of ethics in counselling and psychotherapy* (pp. 50–53). Buckingham, United Kingdom: Open University Press.

PART 4: ETHICS AND THE LAW

4.1 ETHICS AND THE LAW

New Zealand Association of Counsellors. (2002). *Code of ethics*. Hamilton, New Zealand: Author.

Rogers, C. R. (1962). The interpersonal relationship: The core of guidance. *Harvard Educational Review*, 32(4), 416–429.

Further reading

Ludbrook, R. (2003). *Counselling and the law*. Hamilton, New Zealand: New Zealand Association of Counsellors.

4.2 COUNSELLORS AS WITNESSES IN COURT

Feather, R. & Agee, M. (2000). Counsellors as witnesses in Court. *New Zealand Journal of Counselling*, 21(1), 55–75.

New Zealand Association of Counsellors. (2002). *Code of ethics*. Hamilton, New Zealand: Author.

Remley, T. P. J. (1991). *Preparing for court appearances.* Alexandria, VA: American Counseling Association.

Further reading

Ludbrook, R. (2003). *Counselling and the law.* Hamilton, New Zealand: New Zealand Association of Counsellors.

4.3 WHEN A CLIENT GOES TO COURT

Courts 128. (2009). Off to court: Supporting a young witness. Ministry of Justice. Retrieved from http://www.justice.govt.nz/publications/global-publications/o/off-to-court-2013-supporting-a-young-witness-english-courts-128/publication

Courts 129. (2009). Off to court: Being a witness. Ministry of Justice. Retrieved from http://www.justice.govt.nz/publications/global-publications/o/off-to-court-2013-being-a-witness-english-courts-129/publication

Ludbrook, R. (2003). *Counselling and the law.* Hamilton, New Zealand: New Zealand Association of Counsellors.

New Zealand Association of Counsellors. (2002). *Code of ethics.* Hamilton, New Zealand: Author.

4.4 WHEN A COUNSELLOR KNOWS ABOUT ILLEGAL PRACTICES

Agee, M. N. (1997). Privacy and the school counsellor. *Access: Critical perspectives on cultural and policy studies in education, 16*(1), 20–36.

Ludbrook, R. (2003). *Counselling and the law.* Hamilton, New Zealand: New Zealand Association of Counsellors.

New Zealand Association of Counsellors. (2002). *Code of ethics.* Hamilton, New Zealand: Author.

Ponton, R. F. & Duba, J. D. (2009). The ACA Code of Ethics: Articulating counseling's professional covenant. *Journal of Counseling & Development, 87*(1), 117–121.

Futher reading

Simon Jefferson, Ethics and the law, in Part 5, Section 1 of this volume, for a discussion of the duty to warn.

PART 5: WHEN THINGS GO WRONG

INTRODUCTION

Abbott, P. & Wallace, C. (1990). The sociology of the caring professions: An introduction. In P. Abbott & C. Wallace (Eds.), *The sociology of the caring professions* (pp. 1–9). Basingstoke, United Kingdom: Falmer.

Cummings, N. (2008). Foreword. In D. Shapiro, L. Walker, M. Manosevitz, M. Peterson & M. Williams (Eds.), *Surviving a licensing board complaint* (pp. xvii–xix). Pheonix, AZ: Zeig, Tucker, Theisen.

New Zealand Association of Counsellors. (2002). *Code of ethics*. Hamilton, New Zealand: Author.

Ramprogus, V. (1995). *The deconstruction of nursing*. Aldershot, VT: Avebury.

Shapiro, D., Walker, L., Manosevitz, M., Peterson, M. & Williams, M. (2008). *Surviving a licensing board complaint: What to do, what not to do*. Phoenix, AZ: Zeig, Tucker & Theisen.

5.1 WHEN A COLLEAGUE'S PRACTICE IS IMPAIRED

British Association for Counselling and Psychotherapy. (2010). Ethical framework for good practice in counselling and psychotherapy. Author. Retrieved from http://www.bacp.co.uk/ethical_framework/

Clarkson, P. (2001). Responsible involvement: Ethical dimensions of collegial responsibility. In F. P. Barnes & L. Murdin (Eds.), *Values and ethics in the practice of psychotherapy and counselling* (pp. 32–49). Buckingham, United Kingdom: Open University Press.

Corey, G., Corey, M. S. & Callanan, P. (2007). *Issues and ethics in the helping professions* (7th ed.). Belmont, CA: Thomson Brooks/Cole.

New Zealand Association of Counsellors. (2002). *Code of ethics*. Hamilton, New Zealand: Author.

Welfel, E. R. (2010). *Ethics in counselling and psychotherapy: Standards, research, and emerging issues* (4th ed.). Belmont, CA: Brooks/Cole Cengage Learning.

Further reading

American Counseling Association. (2005). Code *of ethics*. http://www.counseling.org/Resources/CodeOfEthics/TP/Home/CT2.aspx

Jones, C., Shillito-Clarke, C., Syme, G., Hill, D., Casemore, R. & Murdin, L. (2000). *Questions of ethics in counselling and therapy*. Buckingham, United Kingdom: Open University Press.

Kottler, J. & Hazler, R. J. (1996). Impaired counselors: The dark side brought into light. *Journal of Humanistic Education and Development, 34*, 98–107.

5.2 TO COMPLAIN OR NOT TO COMPLAIN: THAT IS THE QUESTION

Corey, G. (2009). *Theory and practice of counselling and psychotherapy* (8th ed.). Belmont, CA: Cengage Learning.
Health and Disability Commissioner. (2004). *The code of rights*. Retrieved from http://www.hdc.org.nz/
Hugman, R. (2005). *New approaches in ethics for the caring professions*. Basingstoke, United Kingdom: Palgrave Macmillan.
Manthei, R. & Miller, J. (2000). *Good counselling: A guide for clients*. Auckland, New Zealand: Pearson.
New Zealand Association of Counsellors. (2002). *Code of ethics*. Hamilton, New Zealand: Author.

Further reading

Good counselling: A guide for clients (Manthei & Miller, 2000) provides a readable account by New Zealand authors of how counselling may help and what it may entail. Chapters 10 and 11 on knowing if the help received is appropriate, and what to do if not satisfied, are particularly relevant to this section.

NZAC produces pamphlets at http://www.nzac.org.nz/pamphlets.html that provide some brief basic information about what is likely to happen in counselling and what to do if not satisfied. Those for parents and children may be particularly helpful in clarifying the ethics in this area of work.

NZAC also produces information on the complaints process itself. At http://www.nzac.org.nz/complaints.html there is a flow chart of the process; at http://www.nzac.org.nz/complaints.html a description of the actions NZAC takes when the behaviour complained of warrants a regional educative or restorative approach; and at http://www.nzac.org.nz/raisingconcerns.html there are guidelines for writing a complaint.

5.3 ON BEING A COMPLAINANT

Binmore, K. G. (2005). *Natural justice*. New York: Oxford University Press.
Manthei, R. & Miller, J. (2000). *Good counselling: A guide for clients*. Auckland, New Zealand: Pearson.
New Zealand Association of Counsellors. (2007). Complaints process. Hamilton, New Zealand. Retrieved from http://www.nzac.org.nz/complaints.html
Poppy. (2001). The victim's tale. In R. Casemore (Ed.), *Surviving complaints against counsellors and psychotherapists: Towards understanding and healing* (pp. 1–8). Ross-on-Wye, United Kingdom: PCCS Books.

Further reading

Chapter 11 of *Good counselling: A guide for clients* (Manthei & Miller, 2000) provides a brief perspective on the experience of being a complainant.

'Poppy's' account (see reference above) of her experience as the client of a counsellor, whose behaviour was grossly unethical, evocatively illustrates the difficulty in gaining and maintaining a clear perspective on the service received.

The information on NZAC's website about the association's complaints process offers an overview of how the process works and what is involved from the complainant's perspective. See the website addresses listed in the previous section on whether to complain.

The process undertaken by the Health and Disability Commissioner is described at http://www.hdc.org.nz/complaints/complaints-resolution-overview

5.4 ON BEING A RESPONDENT

'Chris'. (2001). The person complained about was me. In R. Casemore (Ed.), *Surviving complaints against counsellors and psychotherapists: Towards understanding and healing* (pp. 9–17). Ross-on-Wye, United Kingdom: PCCS Books.

Carney, P. (2001). Supervision, support and surviving complaints. In R. Casemore (Ed.), *Surviving complaints against counsellors and psychotherapists: Towards understanding and healing* (pp. 153–160). Ross-on-Wye, United Kingdom: PCCS Books.

Dunnett, A. (2009). The role of the practitioner in self-care in practitioner-client relationship ethics. In L. Gabriel & R. Casemore (Eds.), *Relational ethics in practice: Narratives from counselling and psychotherapy* (pp. 119–130). London, United Kingdom: Routledge.

Jamieson, A. (2001). Surviving a complaint: A practical guide. In *Surviving complaints against counsellors and psychotherapists: Towards understanding and healing* (pp. 19–28). Ross-on-Wye, United Kingdom: PCCS Books.

Paton, I. (2003). If someone complains to NZAC about you: Guidelines for how to respond. *New Zealand Association of Counsellors Newsletter*, 24(1), 15–17.

Schoener, G. R., Milgrom, J. H., Gonsiorek, J. C., Leupker, E. T. & Conroe, R. M. (1989). *Psychotherapists' sexual involvement with clients: Intervention and prevention*. Minneapolis. MN: Walk-In Counseling Center.

Strom-Gottfried, K. (2003). Understanding adjudication: Origins, targets, and outcomes of ethics complaints. *Social Work, 48*(1), 85–95.

Thomas, J. T. (2005). Licensing board complaints: Minimizing the impact on the psychologist's defense and clinical practice. *Professional Psychology: Research and Practice, 36*(4), 426–433.

Welfel, E. R. (2005). Accepting fallibility: A model for personal responsibility for nonegregious ethics infractions. *Counseling and Values, 49*(2), 120–131.
Welfel, E. R. (2010). *Ethics in counselling and psychotherapy: Standards, research, and emerging issues* (4th ed.). Belmont, CA: Brooks/Cole Cengage Learning.
Winslade, J. & White, C. (2002). An analysis of ethics complaints to NZAC: 1991–2000. *New Zealand Journal of Counselling, 23*(2), 1–13.

Further reading

A useful account of being a respondent is contained in chapter 2, 'The person complained about was me' ('Chris', 2001) of a generally excellent edited book, Surviving complaints against counsellors and psychotherapists: Towards understanding and healing.

Chapter 3 (Jamieson, 2001) of the same volume is helpful in providing guidelines for responding to a complaint, and chapter 15 (Carney, 2001) looks at the supervisor's role, if special supervision is required as the result of a complaint.

Recommendations for responding to complaints within the NZAC context are provided by Paton (2003), in an article from the NZAC newsletter which can also be accessed from her website: http://www.perspectives.co.nz/publications.html

A psychologist from the United States, Thomas (2005) – see above – provides a detailed consideration of likely emotional responses to and strategies for addressing complaints.

Chapter 15 on responsibilities for self and colleagues, in Welfel (2010) provides a framework for examining violations of professional ethics. The discussion on how to respond to damage caused is particularly helpful.

5.5 THE NZAC REGIONAL ETHICS PROCESS

New Zealand Association of Counsellors. (2002). *Code of ethics*. Hamilton, New Zealand: Author.

PART 6: EXTENDING ETHICS: THE FUTURE IS ALREADY AT HAND

American Psychological Association. (2009). *Psychology and global climate change: Addressing a multi-faceted phenomenon and set of challenges. A report by the American Psychological Association's task force on the interface between psychology and global climate change* (pp. 1–230). American Psychological

Association. Retrieved from http://www.apa.org/science/about/publications/climate-change.pdf

Benatar, S. R., Daar, A. S. & Singer, P. A. (2005). Global health challenges: The need for an expanded discourse on bioethics. *PLoS Medicine, 2*(7), 0587–0589.

Bosselmann, K. (2001). University and sustainability: Compatible agendas? *Educational Philosophy and Theory, 33*(2), 167–186.

Cornforth, S. C. (2008). Life's span, global warming and ethics: Do counsellors have a part to play in averting a potential catastrophe? *International Journal for the Advancement of Counselling, 30*(3), 145–154.

Fisher, A. (2002). *Radical Ecopsychology: Psychology in the service of life.* Albany, NY: State University of New York Press.

Fisher, M. A. (2009). Replacing "Who is the client?" with a different ethical question. *Professional Psychology: Research and Practice, 40*(1), 1–7.

Furman, G. C. & Gruenewald, D. A. (2004). Expanding the landscape of social justice: A critical ecological analysis. *Educational Administration Quarterly, 40*(1), 47–76.

Gilbert, J. (2005). *Catching the knowledge wave? The knowledge society and the future of education.* Wellington, New Zealand: NZCER Press.

Hung, R. (2007). Is ecological sustainability consonant or dissonant with human rights? Identifying theoretical issues in peace education. *Journal of peace education, 4*(1), 39–55.

Intergovernmental Panel on Climate Change. (2007). *Climate change 2007: Working group II: Impacts, adaption and vulnerability.* Retrieved from http://www.ipcc.ch/publications_and_data/publications_ipcc_fourth_assessment_report_wg2_report_impacts_adaptation_and_vulnerability.htm

Jamieson, D. (2008). *Ethics and the environment.* Cambridge: Cambridge University Press.

Larner, W. & Le Heron, R. (2005). Neo-liberalizing spaces and subjectivities: Reinventing New Zealand universities. *Organization, 12*(6), 843–862.

Leopold, A. (1949). *A sand county almanac.* New York: Oxford University Press.

Metzner, R. (1999). *Green psychology: Transforming our relationship to the earth.* Rochester, VT: Park Street Press.

Naess, A. (1973). The shallow and the deep, long-range ecology movement. A summary. *Inquiry, 16*(1), 95–100.

Naess, A. (1984). A defence of the deep ecology movement. *Environmental Ethics, 6*(3), 265–270.

New Zealand Association of Counsellors. (2002). *Code of ethics.* Hamilton, New Zealand: Author.

O'Neill, J., Holland, A. & Light, A. (2008). *Environmental values.* London, United Kingdom: Routledge.

Paredes, D. M., Choi, K. M., Dipal, M., Edwards-Joseph, A. R., Ermakov, N., Gouveia, A. T., Jain, S., et al. (2008). Globalization: A brief primer for counselors. *International Journal for the Advancement of Counselling, 30*(3), 155–166.

Peters, M. A., Marshall, W. & Webster, S. (Eds.). (1996). *Critical theory, poststructuralism, and the social context.* Palmerston North, New Zealand: Dunmore Press.

Pittock, A. B. (2005). *Climate change.* London, United Kingdom: Earthscan.

Rozak, T. (1999). Foreword. In *Green psychology: Transforming our relationship to the earth* (pp. viii-x). Rochester, VT: Park Street Press.

Sevenhuijsen, S. (1998). *Citizenship and the ethics of care: Feminist considerations on justice, morality, and politics.* New York: Routledge.

Shepard, P. (1982). *Nature and madness.* San Francisco, CA: Sierra Club Books.

Singer, P. (2002). *Animal liberation.* New York: Ecco.

Sliep, Y. & Kotze, E. (2007). Weaving a learning community by the telling, deconstructing and retelling of life stories. In K. Maree (Ed.), *Shaping the story: A guide to facilitating narrative counselling* (pp. 138–151). Pretoria, South Africa: Van Schaik.

Sterba, J. P. (2001). *Three challenges to ethics.* New York: Oxford University Press.

INDEX

ABOUT THE CONTRIBUTORS

Editors

Kathie Crocket, PhD, is Director of Counsellor Education at the University of Waikato. She is a member of the NZAC National Ethics Committee, and has served on the University's Faculty of Education Research Ethics Committee.

Margaret Agee, PhD, leads the Counsellor Education Programme at the University of Auckland. She is a member of the NZAC National Ethics Committee, and has written articles and facilitated training events on aspects of ethical practice.

Sue Cornforth, PhD, lectures in reflexive practice and social and environmental justice in educational contexts at Victoria University of Wellington (VUW). She co-chairs the Faculty of Education Ethics Committee at VUW, and has a longstanding interest in counsellor education as well as experience in counselling practice.

Contributors

Alastair Crocket, EdD, is a Principal Academic Staff Member at Waikato Institute of Technology. His doctoral thesis explored Pakeha counsellors' experiences of practising with people from other cultures. Alastair represents Waikato/Bay of Plenty on NZAC National Executive.

Philip Culbertson, PhD, is a writer and lecturer affiliated with the University of Auckland and the College of the Desert in Palm Springs, California. In addition to writing and teaching, he worked in Auckland for nine years as a psychotherapist in private practice while teaching Social and Cultural Issues in Psychotherapy at AUT.

Jim Depree, MCouns, PGDipSocWork, BA, works part-time as a counsellor in private practice and part-time as a Family Engagement Worker for the Napier CYF Supervised Group Home. He is also working part-time on a PhD at Waikato University, "Taping for therapeutic purposes in couple therapy". He is a member of the NZAC Regional Ethics Team.

Ireni Esler BEd. BSocAdmin, DipT, is currently completing a doctorate on counselling supervision and will then take a sabbatical from her independent private practice to travel the world. Ireni spent nearly ten years on the NZAC's Ethics Committee, three of those in her capacity as Auckland Regional Representative on National Executive. Ireni was part of the consultative group that revised the *Code of Ethics* in 2002.

Carol Fatialofa (Meredith), BA, DipGuidCouns, is of Samoan-Chinese and Samoan-English heritage. For more than 20 years, Carol has worked in the fields of career and employment guidance and counselling, counselling supervision, training, mentoring and education. She contributed to the book *Penina Uliuli: Contemporary Challenges in Mental Health for Pacific Peoples* (2007, University of Hawai'i Press).

Rachael Feather, MEd(Couns) is a Registered Psychotherapist in private practice, currently completing her training in Jungian Psychoanalysis through ANZSJA CGJI. For her masters research, Rachael investigated the experiences of counsellors who had served as factual witnesses in legal processes. She was a member of the NZAC Ethics Review Committee from 2000-2002.

Kaaren Frater-Mathieson, MEd(Couns) works part-time in private practice as a counsellor, supervisor and professional development trainer, and part-time as a writer. For many years she worked with refugee survivors of trauma. She was a senior tutor for the Counsellor Education programme at the University of Auckland, and took part in contract research into refugee education for the Ministry of Education, contributing to the book, *Educational Interventions for Refugee Children* (RoutledgeFalmer).

Bill Grant, MNZAP (Advanced Clinical Practice), Registered Psychotherapist, also maintains his membership in NZAC. He is currently Clinical Advisor, Sensitive Claims Unit, ACC, Wellington. He previously worked in the Department of Psychological Medicine at Wakari and Dunedin Hospitals; in the Department of Education, University of Otago; as a Visiting Guidance Counsellor in the Ministry of Education; as Ethics Secretary for the NZAC; and for ten years in private practice.

Colin Hughes, PGDipCouns, BA(Hons), TTC, AdvCertSupervision, is Head of Guidance at Trident High School, Whakatane. His professional interests and experience include supervision, Myers Briggs, and counselling adolescents. He served for eight years on the NZAC National Ethics Committee, and four years as Regional Ethics Coordinator for Waikato/Bay of Plenty.

Simon Jefferson, Barrister, has been legal advisor to NZAC for twenty years. He has led many training events for NZAC and counsellor education programmes, as well as for the Law Society, and he has contributed comment on topical legal issues in NZAC Newsletters. He is a specialist in family law.

Hyeeun Kim, MEd(Couns), MTheol, ThM, BA, MNZAC, originally from Korea, is a counsellor and clinical supervisor in Auckland. She is also an ordained minister of the Presbyterian Church of Aotearoa New Zealand and the Presbyterian Church of Korea She has been a committee member of The Asian Network Inc., East Health (PHO) and Korean Community Wellness Inc. Her PhD research at the University of Auckland explores the parenting experiences of 1.5 generation Korean-Kiwis.

Professor Bob Manthei, was a counsellor educator at the University of Canterbury for 34 years before retiring in 2008. He has been a member of NZAC since 1974, is a Life Member, and currently serves on the Canterbury-Westland Branch Committee. He continues to research and write about counselling outcome and practice.

Antony McFelin, BTheol, MEd, Executive Officer, NZAC, has been involved with NZAC since 1997 and during this time has served as a President of the Association. Antony's contribution to this book reflects his interest in queer issues for counsellors from his position of life as a gay man.

Eric Medcalf, BA(Hons), CertApplSocSci, CQSW, DipPsychotherapy, MNZAP (ACP), Registered Psychotherapist, also maintains his NZAC membership. Based in Wellington until 2010, he is currently on sabbatical in New York City. He was previously Convenor of the NZAC Ethics Committee and a member of the Council of NZAP. Eric is a World Music radio presenter.

Carl Mika, a lecturer in the Department of Policy, Culture and Social Sciences in Education at the University of Waikato, has a background in law, Indigenous and Māori Studies, and teaches in the areas of educational philosophy, social justice and education, Māori issues and education, and indigenous and postcolonial studies. He is a member of the Faculty of

Education Research Ethics Committee. His current PhD study explores the works of the German romantic poet and philosopher Novalis, and applies his philosophies to a Māori theory of language and Being. Karl's tribal affiliations are Tuhourangi and Ngati Whanaunga.

Judi Miller, PhD, is an Associate Professor in the Health Sciences Centre in the College of Education at the University of Canterbury, where she has been teaching for 22 years. She co-ordinates the solution-focused counselling programme. Her interests include exploring how to ensure that brief therapy is effective, the impact of meaningful alliances on counselling outcomes, and the professionalisation of counselling in Aotearoa New Zealand.

Fran Parkin, MCouns, BA, PTSTA, is a counsellor, psychotherapist, and supervisor who for many years combined her work in private practice with teaching and lecturing. Fran currently works full-time as part of a group counselling and psychotherapy practice in Wellington.

Rhonda Pritchard, BA(Hons), BSocSc, DipTchg, CTA, MNZAC, MNZPsS, from Wellington, was in practice as a counsellor, supervisor, trainer and mediator for twenty-nine years and was Convenor of the Ethics Committee of NZAC from 2003–06. In 2007 she joined the Ministry of Social Development as a researcher on homicide in families, and was later appointed a Member of the New Zealand Parole Board. Her publications include: *Love in the Real World: Starting and keeping close relationships* and *Children are Unbeatable: 7 very good reasons not to hit children.*

Jenny Snowdon, MCouns, is currently a resident of Hamilton. Her work includes counselling in homes, providing teaching support for the counsellor education programmes at the University of Waikato and Wintec, and supervision. Her interest in ethics began in earnest when she majored in philosophy in her undergraduate degree.

Candy Vong, MEd(Couns), originally from Macau, China, is an experienced Asian ACC-approved counsellor, supervisor and trainer working in the Health and Counselling Service at the University of Auckland and in private practice. She provides psychological interventions for several PHOs, is a trustee and practitioner with the Chinese Mental Health Consultation Service, and facilitates presentations and training events for professional organisations and the wider community.

Sue Webb, MPhil, BA(Hons), BEd(Couns), PGCE is a counselling consultant in private practice in Palmerston North, having previously lectured for twenty-nine years in counselling at Massey University. She was one of two National Executive Liaison representatives on the NZAC Ethics Committee when it was first set up in 1994 and, after a period as NZAC President, returned to the Ethics Committee in 2001, where she is presently the Convenor. Sue is Secretary on the Executive Council of the International Association of Counselling.

Joy Te Wiata, MCouns, is a Rangatira Kaimahi, clinical co-leader and therapist in Te Kakano at SAFE Network. Her connection to SAFE began in 2005 with SAFE Overseas Services, working on Pitcairn Island. Joy worked several years for Toiora Whanau, her iwi social service team in the Manawatu/Horowhenua region. Her iwi affiliations are Ngati Raukawa.

John Winslade, PhD, is a part time Associate Professor at the University of Waikato and also a Professor and Associate Dean at California State University San Bernardino. He twice chaired the committee that revised the NZAC *Code of Ethics* and was a member of the NZAC Ethics Committee from 1994-2003, including five years as its convenor.

Carol White, PGCertCounsSup DipEdGuid, DipPE, DipT, Life Member NZAC, contributed to the development of the first NZAC *Code of Ethics* and to rewriting the current Code. A past president of NZAC, she has been a member of the National Ethics Committee since 2000. Until recently a counsellor with management responsibilities at the University of Auckland, she is currently a consultant and private practitioner.

Vi Woolf is of Ngati Whatua and Ngapuhi descent, and is in private practice in South Auckland. She specialises in cultural mentoring and is currently serving on the Membership Committee of NZAC. On the NZAC National Executive Vi holds the position of Te Ahi Kaa.

Jeannie Wright, PhD, Associate Professor of Counselling, is based at Massey University's Hokowhitu campus in Palmerston North. She migrated to Aotearoa in 2006 and has been a member of NZAC since 2007. She is a senior accredited member of the British Association for Counselling and Psychotherapy and has taught ethics, both in practice settings and for research.